Burn Fat Fast Through The Revolutionary

Ten UP System™

William Scannell and Michele Blood

Copyright © W. Scannell & M. Blood

May 2015

MusiVation International Publishing

MusiVation International LLC

P O Box 12933

La Jolla California 92039

USA

Printed in the United States of America

ISBN#: 978-1-890679-05-7

Call 1 (858) 268-8688 for wholesale copies of paperback and audio book versions or email MusiVation@aol.com

Cover Design by M. Blood & T. Rogers Cartoons by Sanjay and M. Blood Photographs by W. Scannell

Burn Fat Fast Through The Revolutionary Ten UP System™

Become Your Perfect Weight

Looking Good & Feeling Great

Even When Sleeping

William Scannell & Michele Blood

Disclaimer

The information in this book is not intended or implied to be a substitute for professional medical advice, diagnosis or treatment.

All content including text, graphics, images and information contained on or available through this book is for general information purposes only. We accept no responsibility for the accuracy of information contained on or available throughout this book and such information is subject to change without notice.

While energy, psychology, and mind body treatments have produced excellent clinical results and are constantly gaining scientific support daily they are still unfortunately, not widely accepted as a formally validated scientific technique.

Members of the public must therefore take complete responsibility for their own use of energy and mind body techniques.

DEDICATION

This book and all the information within, is dedicated to you, the reader, and only you. As of this moment, there is nothing else except you and your mind. This book is for you and about you. We wrote it for you and not for us, as we already know this Ten UP System™ works!

This information can transform your life. If you are someone who feels trapped in your life and cannot find a way forward to achieve what you want, then this book is for you. This knowledge will benefit you in every detail of your life. From this day forward, when you take action. Everything is possible!

The only thing that is standing between you, the body you want, and the life you would like, is a little knowledge and a new awareness. This book is about awakening your awareness.

Awareness is everything!

You can apply the information in this book to everything and anything in your life.

Even if you are using a weight release system right now and getting results, by applying some of the techniques in this book, you will turbo charge your health, feel a little brighter, and lighter every single day. Take a deep breath, exhale slowly, and enjoy.

Here's to your new life and your new body!

William & Michele

ABOUT THE AUTHORS

Michele Blood

Michele Blood is a successful, multi-talented person with a diverse business arena. In addition to creating MusiVation™ products and seminars worldwide, she has also trained major companies worldwide. Her public Mystical and Success Events have been held in over fourteen countries. Her largest audience was fifty thousand in Kuala Lumpur. She has written and produced over one hundred products and seminars including books, audio programs, music CD's, Infomercial's, DVD Training Systems and videos. Michele has co-authored some of these books and products with well-known speakers including five programs with Bob Proctor and a co-authored book with Bob Proctor titled "Become A Magnet To Money Through The Sea Of Unlimited Consciousness".

Michele experienced a spiritual awakening several years ago. She is now dedicated to assisting others to awaken and grow in higher consciousness, to experience true health, in body, mind and spirit. To do this Michele started The Mystical Success Club™, (www.MysticalSuccessClub.com) which now has members in over twenty-four countries. The members are enjoying more success, love, joy, peace and higher spiritual consciousness.

Brian Tracy, bestselling author comments, *"Michele has put together materials that bring about permanent behavioral change."*

William Scannell

William Scannell hails from Ireland. He has experienced many achievements in his life, including, running a successful import business, winning numerous competitions in many different sports, including boxing.

After experiencing a knee injury William discovered a way to keep fit and healthy while he was healing. He began to train adults and children who were overweight with his new method, and with outstanding results. These adults and children, in no time at all, were releasing weight fast, due to Williams Ten UP System™.

William realized that he felt happiest when helping others accomplish their physical goals, especially with these children, when nobody else believed in them, William did and guided them to health and happiness.

Today he teaches his Ten UP System™ relaxation and meditation classes and is fully committed to assisting others to find happiness, higher consciousness and physical health.

www.WilliamScannell.com

Table of Contents

Dedication..iv

About The Authors.....................................v

Introduction...1

No Pills No Shakes.....................................3

Knowledge And Information.......................5

Your New Mantra......................................6

No More Excuses......................................10

Trust In Life & Learn To Live....................11

Things Are Not Always What They Seem....15

More Than Burning Fat Fast......................18

Awareness...20

Wake Up To Life.......................................24

Here's Cheers To H2o...............................26

How It Works...34

Get Moving..36

Visualization..38

The Rope And Centrifugal Force...............45

The Ten Up System™................................46

The Five-Minute System..........................56

The Music..58

How To Make The Ten Up System™ Skipping Rope.......62

The Key To Your Success..........................81

Conscious And Sub-Conscious Alignment....83

What Foods To Eat...................................85

Table of Contents continued

What Not To Eat 97

Short Term Stress Busters 102

Foods That Calm Your Mind 104

A Good Night's Sleep 105

Simple & Easy Ways To Reduce Fat 107

Belly Fat And Lower Back Pain 114

12 Minute Abs Workout 118

Affirmations 121

Goal Setting 129

The Magnetic Future Self Board 134

Your Daily Action List 138

The Power Of Meditation 143

Love And Gratitude 148

Putting It All Together 150

Pages To Write Your Goals And Intentions 156

INTRODUCTION

This book started out for the sole purpose of William wishing to supply one person with the knowledge of how to burn or release fat easily.

At the time, when he spoke about this subject to just one person at a time he simply shared the experience that he had discovered. He found people where burning fat FAST! To his surprise, everyone that heard about his Ten UP System™ wanted to know more.

William met Michele Blood after he had become part of her Mystical Success Club™ and Michele suggested that William write a book.

Michele encouraged William and helped him to understand that many people in the world need to know what he knew, as millions of people struggle with fat every day and do not know what to do about this problem. These people needed good, honest information that works.

Michele and William then made a decision to add both of their expertise and write the book together.

The best part about this system is that you do not even have to leave your home.

Neither Michele nor William claim to be experts, they simply have the experience and have assisted others and know this Ten UP System™ works. Unfortunately, many of the self-proclaimed experts do not have enough knowledge to help you, but they do know that they can easily mislead you on any subject that has struggle attached to it.

If you apply the knowledge that is in this book, then you will do exactly what it says on the cover: "Burn Fat Fast" and so much more.

Please read this book slowly from cover to cover, as these ideas may be quite new to some of you. Keep an open mind and you will BECOME YOUR PERFECT WEIGHT LOOKING GOOD AND FEELING GREAT!

Once you have read this book in its entirety, perhaps put it aside and go for a walk. As you walk, pay attention to where you mind wanders but more importantly pay attention to what your mind is doing.

Relax your mind, perhaps you can sit in your favorite cafe and allow your mind to absorb this new information, because this is all about you and your mind. This knowledge will change your life.

After reading this book, you may find you begin to look at the world a little differently. So please, just allow it to be as simple as that and enjoy the journey.

NO NEED TO LEAVE YOUR HOME

NO PILLS

NO SHAKES

NO EXPENSIVE BULKY EQUIPMENT

The Ten UP System™ Works!

With the Ten UP System™, you will find the latest in positive mind technology that is available today. With this system, you can release fat, and as much as you want, however the most vital and significant message is teaching you how to keep it off.

The mind technology chapters help remove the stubborn habitude of unconscious behavior that has been holding you back.

Why Don't They Teach This In Schools

We know that by the end of this book, you will ask yourself the following question: Why don't they teach this in schools?

We want people to take this information and use it. We would like everyone to share these new ideas, for there are great rewards in helping other people.

We also know, that you will become more aware of what your children are being exposed to in school, and at home.

We will make you the star of your life. How will we teach you this? We will teach you the fun way.

We have confidence that some of this vital information will eventually be taught in schools.

Knowledge and Information

From this moment forward, you will have to release all of the information and knowledge that you have learned over the years, information and knowledge that has been holding you back.

The Information and knowledge that we are referring to, is what you have read in magazines, heard from certain nutritionists, doctors and on television programs.

The information in this book has always been available but you were simply unaware of it, until now.

We are not going to talk about Hormones, Insulin Levels or Leptin, as others tend to do.

If these things really worked, then why is there such a big problem in the world today with too much unhealthy fat?

Just look around and see all the people that are struggling with excess fat. How many people do you know that have a flat stomach? How many people do you know that are happy with their body?

OK YOU ASKED FOR IT

ALMOST EVERYTHING THAT THE DIET INDUSTRY AND SO MANY OTHERS TELL YOU IS ABSOLUTE BULLSHIT!

This is simply because these so call experts' do not really know what works and are solely interested in hiking their sales figures. People are being taught, the exact reverse of what works.

TAKE THIS JOURNEY AND CLEAN OUT YOUR MIND OF ALL THAT MIS-INFORMATION THAT YOU HAVE ABSORBED AND BEEN CONDITIONED TO BELIEVE OVER THE YEARS.

YOUR NEW MANTRA

I AM NOW AT MY PERFECT WEIGHT LOOKING GOOD AND FEELING GREAT!

TODAY I HAVE A BRAND NEW LIFE.
I AM HEALTHY, HAPPY, & FIT
I AM OVER FLOWING WITH POSITIVE ENERGY.
I AM ENERGY!

JUST KEEP SAYING and SINGING THESE POWERFUL THOUGHTS AND SEE WHAT HAPPENS NEXT

One year and even one month from today, you will be so happy that you started. This moment is all you have. Live in every moment fully.

PS To further assist these powerful words entering your sub-conscious mind fast, Michele has some of her MusiVation™ affirmation songs as a gift with the purchase of this book. The powerful affirmations enter your sub-conscious mind 300 times faster with music, than just saying them aloud.

Go to this link to receive these two powerful mind-changing songs as a FREE GIFT. Enjoy...

http://www.musivation.com/TenUpFreeGift.html

WITH PERSISTENCE
YOU CAN DEFEAT ALL OBSTACLES

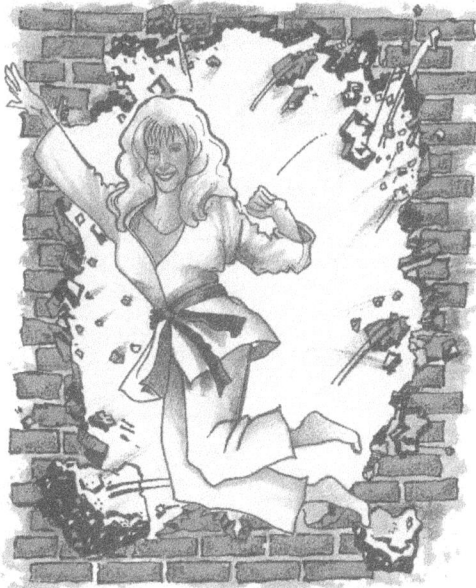

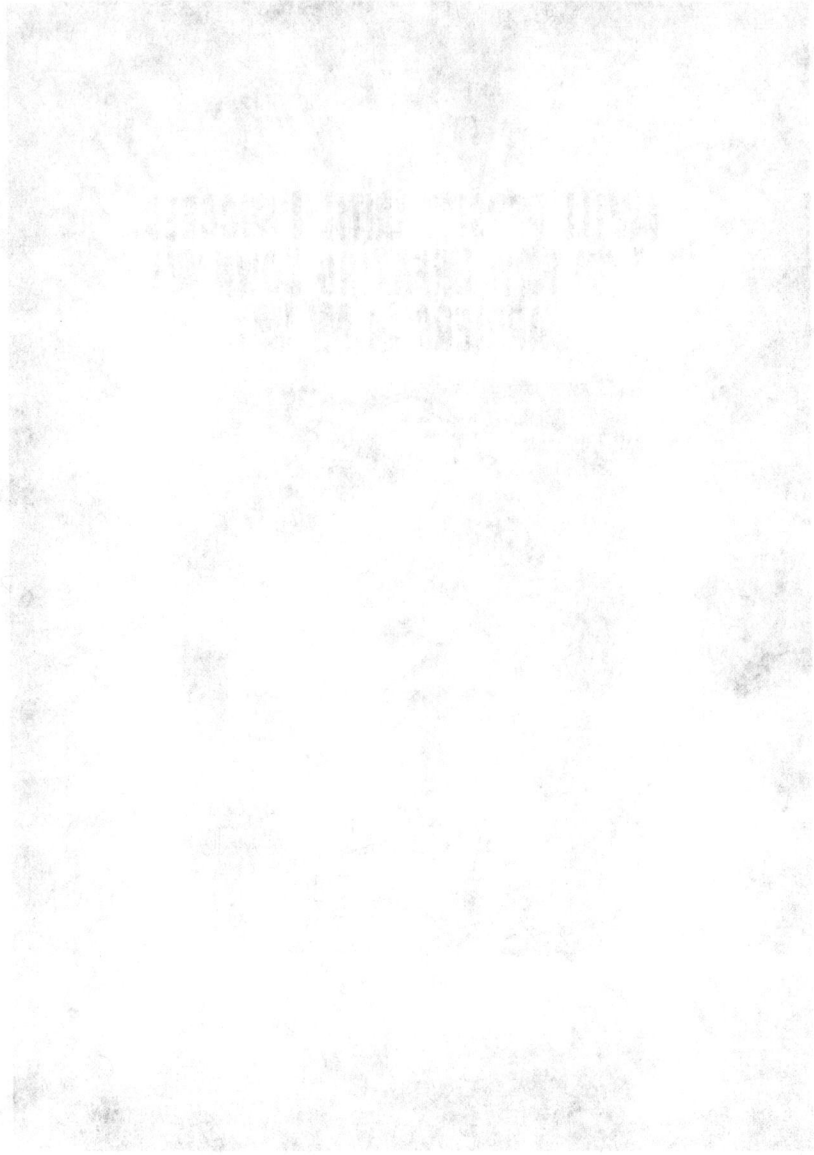

AGREEMENT

Before you start, we would like you agree to accept the information that is in this book, as this will change your life.

If you agree to this, please sign below.

I _____,

AGREE TO BEGIN A NEW LIFE. A LIFE OF HEALTH, POSITIVE THINKING AND TO ACHIEVE MY PERFECT WEIGHT LOOKING GOOD AND FEELING GREAT!

Date: _____

Welcome to your new life.

Today is your day, your day to finally release the fat that you have been storing and regain control of your life.

From this moment on, you are taking back your life.

NO MORE EXCUSES

Today you are going to take 100% responsibility for your life.

No more blaming someone else or any situation for where you are now. You are going to take responsibility for looking good and feeling great! Once you learn to do this, you will progress so much faster.

If you accept that you have created where you are right now, then you can accept that you can create something much better, and that you can let go and let your past be in the past forever.

What would you attempt in your life today, if you knew you could not fail?

You would feel wonderful. Yes, you would and you will.

As you go forward from here, you are going to reshape your life, into the life you have always wanted. Right now, your mind is so full of misinformation that it is like a garden full of weeds. By reading and taking action from the advice in this book, you have decided to plant seeds of a beautiful fruit tree in your new healthy garden.

As you go forward from here, each page that you read will be picking the weeds from your garden/sub-conscious mind and at the same time, planting the seeds for your new life.

By the end of this book, you will have planted the seeds for your new future. Then your only job is to water those seeds and wait for them to grow into beautiful, fruit filled trees. There will be no going back to that place where you felt trapped in a body you knew was not the real you.

TRUST IN LIFE & LEARN TO LIVE
STOP TAKING LIFE SO SERIOUSLY
GIVE YOURSELF A BREAK FROM STRESS
AND HAVE FUN IN YOUR LIFE

The world is full of people who take life so seriously. Take a break from the worlds seriously unhappy people. They do not need your membership into their game of misery any longer. You certainly do not want to catch what they have.

You will not be missed. Go ahead and release the negative gossiping complainers from your life. Do it for a month. If the rest of the world misses you, you can always go back.

One of the biggest lessons in life to remember is that we all have FREE WILL. We can make our own decisions and choices. We do not have to follow the masses.

You will hear people say that everyone has free will, but people really do not understand what this means and do not know how to achieve it. Some people choose to live their life by complaining about everything.

Other people just choose to live.

We can choose where and what we want to be, because everything has two sides. All we have to do is move to the other side. Laugh as much as you can and create time for joy in your life.

You can always find good reasons to smile and be grateful. Think of someone or something that makes you smile. Focus your mind on happy things and happy experiences.

Add humor to your days, and look at the funny side of life.

11

When we start to look at life with joy and not take it all so seriously, a funny thing begins to shift. We actually begin to see things that were always there, but somehow were invisible before. This is because we were taking life too seriously and complaining. When we complain we block the joy that life has to offer. Here are a few examples:

- Do you complain about things that you can do nothing about?

- Do you complain about the weather to your friends?

- Do you complain about money and the banking system to your friends?

- Do you complain about other people you do not even know?

Please read very carefully. Complaining is a complete waste of energy. YOUR energy. We are all either gaining or losing energy and complaining is one of the most powerful ways to lose...well...YOUR POWER.

The next five people that you meet during your day please pay special attention to what they are saying. Are they complementing someone, is it good news that they are sharing, is it a happy conversation? Probably not.

Try to distance yourself from people that are always complaining because they are draining your power and your life energy.

This is your energy and you need every bit of it to feel happy and to release fat and begin a new life.

When we begin to gain energy, we raise our vibration and we begin to have a higher awareness of the beautiful life that has been waiting all along. We must be open and receptive to better life experiences. As we become more aware, we also become much happier. Sometimes what we need is right there in front of us, but we are unable to see it. We are unable to see it because we are wasting our life force on negative energies that we do not resonate with, and that often make us depressed. These distractions can easily be a bad influence and lower our consciousness.

We are so busy focusing our attention on something or somewhere else that we have unconsciously created a blind spot in our life. These blind spots stop us in our tracks from seeing what is right there waiting in front of us. The wonderful, happy, supportive people, opportunities, joy and beauty.

Here is a little humor to explain it.

One morning a man, who did not believe in anything, awoke from a dream and claimed that God had spoken to him. He alleged that God said to him, *I will show you my power and that I exist.*

Everyone thought this man had lost his mind as he danced around the streets shouting that there is a God and that he was going to show him His power. The man noticed that people were not taking him seriously, so he decided that he would prove it to them. He told them that he was going to jump into the ocean and that God would come to save him. He started to swim out to sea, until he had no energy left and no way back.

As he waited in the sea, treading water, a ship came along and offered to save him, but he refused to board it, explaining that he was waiting for God to show up. An hour later, another ship sailed by and tried to help, but he told them the same thing. He now began to tire, and was finding it a problem staying afloat. At that exact moment, a very big cruise liner showed up and tried to rescue him, but once again, he told them that God would save him.

As the current got stronger, he noticed a lifeboat, which must have broken away from a ship, drifting past him. He grabbed the lifeboat and hoisted himself up to look inside.

The boat was fully equipped with food, blankets and a first aid kit. He considering entering but decided against it, reasoning with himself that God was going to save him.

One hour later, he drowned.

When he arrived in heaven, he asked God angrily why he had not saved him. God looked at him and said *what are you doing here? I sent you three ships and a lifeboat.*

Things Are Not Always What They Seem

What we are looking for in life may show up in ways we never could have imagined.

An Example:

William remembers one time coming back from a buying trip to Indonesia and Thailand and discovering that he had overspent by forty thousand dollars.

He was worried because he was approaching the quietest time of the year and he had staff to pay, high rent bills and so on. *(William owned a beautiful store in Ireland and bought from the indigenous people their hand made furniture and hand crafted items. He did this directly and paid them much more than large wholesalers to help these beautiful people make decent money and feed their families.)*

A new friend entered Williams' life who had a business nearby. He called William in to welcome him back from his trip. William explained that he had gone a bit overboard on his last buying trip and that he had no idea where he was going to find the extra money.

A sum of money that size takes time to secure and he had several forty-foot shipping containers on the way from Indonesia and Thailand. William did not expect him to offer any suggestions, as he was a very quiet person.

William had spent all day thinking about this challenge and possible solutions.

That night, as William lay awake in bed, his head began to throb from thinking of any solution to his so-called problem.

The next morning William arrived to his store at 9.30am. While in the process of opening the doors and disarming the alarm, this new friend drove up and beckoned him to his car. He asked William to get in and join him. This was a very new acquaintance and both knew very little about each other.

What happened next was something that William would never have imagined even if he were to think of every possible outcome to his so-called problem.

When William sat in his car, he asked his new friend how he was. His new friend did not respond to this question but simply said, *"Here is an envelope with $30,000 within. Pay me back when you can"*.

William was stunned. If it were not for that white envelope, William would have thought that he was dreaming. William gratefully accepted this money and paid his new friend back quickly.

William realized that after looking for all possible solutions, he would never have imagined such kindness.

So please be open and receptive to life and be willing to receive and give and all good will come to you. We must be open and receptive to change. Change comes from within. Open your mind and heart to changing your life. All of this will make more and more sense as you read. Changing your body requires an openness to receive and give.

We suggest you begin your new life quietly. In other words, do not listen to what others have to say. This is your life and we know that you can change the feeling of being not in control of your life or weight. You can live a life of joy and freedom.

Once you release the old negative self-talk and old mind programs, the fat will also begin to melt away.

Why would anyone try to stop you from improving your life?

Think about it.

In the end, we only regret the things that we did not do.

Do not let negative people live in your head.
Just kick them out.

MORE THAN BURNING FAT FAST

The burn fat fast method is so much more than just releasing fat. It is true self-discovery so that you can start looking within for the solution and not without.

We will use the outside method to remove the fat first and then we will teach you how to go inside to keep it off permanently, without the struggle.

This book is all about you, and no one else. It is only about you. Please remember that. Do not worry about what other people think or say. Your thoughts and opinions are the only ones that matter. What other people think is none of our business and most people are only thinking of themselves anyway!

The point of this book, is for you to reach the realization that you can do anything you want, once you quiet the mind, and all that crazy mind chatter.

The benefits in your life will be very surprising and for some will feel miraculous.

As mentioned previously in this book, slowly integrate these ideas into your daily life. This way you will get wonderful results, which will affect your life and not only in the fat removal area.

This is your handbook for life!

The Ten UP System™ is so easy to learn, and the other chapters in this book will be simple, fun and easy to learn as well as to implement every day.

The information in this book will be of great benefit to you. It will help you look and feel better about yourself. You will gain more confidence and clarity. Once you master this method, you <u>will not</u> need a coach, nutritionists or even a gym. Now that is not to say you cannot go to a gym. Gyms can be fun, and fun is so important in life.

So many people see things they would like to do, but then when they read words like commitment follow a program or invest in yourself, scary words for most, fears pop up. We trust that by the end of this book, you will understand what your fears are and how to release your fears and let go of your old paradigms of low self-esteem and of course fat. You will look at fear in a different way.

FEAR
False Evidence Appearing Real

The only thing that stands in the way of you achieving your dreams is your old way of thinking, in other words, your mind.

With the information in this book, you can make your own program that suits you. What is on offer here is for you to eat the food that we suggest and stay away from some of the foods that have been destroying your chances of achieving the body you desire. How easy is that?

You do not have to work on this, but it would be great if you wanted to. That would be enough for you to get what you want.

What we share in this book is the easiest way.

By using the simple advice in this book, let today be the first day on your journey to the new you.

AWARENESS

Awareness is one of the most important things that you can develop in your life right now.

**The definition of insanity is...
doing the same things repeatedly and expecting a different result.**

Without awareness, you are like a machine expecting different results and that is frankly CRAZY!

The message in this book is mainly about awareness. If you have been struggling with body fat, and tried numerous systems with little results, it is because of your lack of awareness.

Up until now, you were unaware of this information.

We can help you with this.

Believe us when we say, that by the end of this book you will have a more heightened awareness than you ever had before and not just in the fat removal area.

History books tell us about how America was discovered and by whom, but the odd thing about this statement is that the land of America was always there and the people as well.

Prior to the arrival of Leif Erikson and Christopher Columbus, America as we now know it, was already inhabited by people who walked, and hunted, and lived their lives, just as their fathers and forefathers had before them, and they were aware that they existed.

Try to tell them, that they did not exist.

America as we now know it existed, but the Europeans were simply unaware of it.

It was not in their awareness.

Some people became very rich when they discovered oil on their land. The oil was always there, even before they were born. They were just not aware of it.

Picture this, you are playing cards with a group of people, and when you have a good hand, no one will bet, but when they do bet, they always win.

You think that you are just having bad luck because every hand you have is beaten.

Everyone takes a break for fifteen minutes and two strangers introduce themselves to you in the hallway.

The two strangers that you met in the hallway told you that there is a mirror positioned behind your head, and because of this, everyone can see your cards, and that is the reason why no one will play when you have a good hand.

When you return to the table, you now see the mirror hanging on the wall behind your seat. Your knowledge of the mirror will change the outcome of the game from that moment forward because of your new awareness.

We are these strangers in the hallway and we will show you what is holding you back and help you accomplish what you want to achieve in your life whether it be fat removal or anything else.

The following is an example of a person, with a good sense of awareness.

Have you ever heard of an airline called Ryanair? Ryanair is the third largest airline in Europe today and it grew very fast in a short period all because they employed one unique man. Even during the recession when all of the other airlines were losing money, he was still making profits and buying new aircraft. He was making more money than ever before.

In 2012, the airline carried 79.6 million passengers, and had a fleet of 305 aircraft. This airline started as a family run business.

To get to the point;

This unique person is Michael O'Leary and in 1994, he became the chief executive officer of Ryanair Ireland. His estimated net worth in 2012, was in the region of four hundred million Euro.

In Dublin, hundreds of thousands of car owners hit the roads every morning on their way to work. Due to congestion, traffic would be at standstill for long periods and the masses would sit in their cars complaining about the traffic problem.

In Dublin city, like most major cities, there are specific traffic lanes, for buses and taxis that enable them to move freely.

Michael does not sit in traffic like the masses because he has a higher awareness.

What he did was register his car as a taxi by buying a taxi plate for his Mercedes. He then had a meter installed to classify it as a taxi so he could legally zip down Dublin's bus lanes and speed his progress around the city.

What makes him different to the masses here? He has a higher awareness.

When he decides to advertise his company, he does not hire expensive advertising companies to run advertisements for him on the TV, radio stations and newspapers all over Europe. His mind does not think that way.

He looks at it in a creative way and asks himself, how do I get twenty million worth of free advertising? He does not see a reason why he should pay for this.

When he wants twenty million euro worth of advertising in Europe without paying for it, what does he do? He just tells a reporter that he has asked Boeing to remove all but one toilet from his planes so he can put in more seats, and that he will charge people £1 to use the one toilet that is left. Then he will say with the toilets gone he will fit more people on each flight, which in turn lowers the price of the flight for everyone and that makes the customers happy.

The following month he will say that he is introducing standing in his plane to be able to get more people on board like a bus, and that he is doing this for the customers as they will pay less if they are standing.

Many years ago, he said he was going to add a Fat Tax and that he would weigh customers at check in. Many airlines today are trying to copy him.

The media jump on these stories claiming that he was insane and every newspaper in Europe was running these stories on the front page. Even the radio stations are talking about him and his low cost airline. They are all arguing and questioning if it is a good idea or bad for fliers.

He just got about 20 million euros worth of advertising free, when everyone else is paying top dollar for it.

He is famous for saying.

WHAT PART OF NO REFUND, DON'T YOU
UNDERSTAND?

Whether we agree with his tactics is not the point. Awareness is the key.

WAKE UP TO LIFE
Stop walking as slowly and as carefully as you can to death.

Here you receive the gift of your life. Most people's awareness lever is set to the switched off position and they live 90% of their lives in the past, recalling stories of yesterday and remaining 9% in the future talking about what they would like in their lives however, they have no idea how to achieve what they want.

When you have all of this mind chatter going on in your head, how is it possible to be aware of anything? The first thing you need to do is stop watching the news and reading the newspapers, unless your job depends on it. The information that comes from these sources is normally rubbish that makes your poor mind a bowl of mush and nine times out of ten it is useless data.

If anything important comes up, one of your friends or relatives is bound to share it with you. When we say important, we mean something that directly affects you and your everyday life and not what some celebrity said or did.

These celebrities do not know you so why should you care about what clothes they are wearing, who are they dating and other useless information that clutters the mind.

You can be the star in your own life, but instead, you have become part of the audience just looking in.

How absurd is that.

Everything you need in your life exists at this moment but it is just not in your awareness field right now. That is why you are unaware of it.

You focus on what other people are doing and saying, and as a result, you have forgotten about living your own life.

If you are sitting down watching the TV soaps and following celebrities' lives, then my friend, you are dead. The funny thing here is you do not even know it. One day, you will look back at your life and wonder where all the time went. You will ask yourself where your life went. Did you use your precious life up sitting in front of the TV?

A well-known person once said that the meaning of life was to raise a family. If you have children then it is your job to love and rear them, but that is not all that there is to life. You have the right to live your life too. Do not identify yourself with just rearing children. You are so much more than that, a person with endless possibilities. You are unique in every way, one of a kind, with unique hidden gifts. At this moment, you are simply unaware of them because you have been programmed, from a very young age, to stay within the confines of the pack.

Until NOW!

HERE'S CHEERS TO H2O

The Miracle Of Water

In this book, we will continuously remind you, to drink a LOT of water.

Before you start this system, we recommend that you consult your doctor to see if you are ready for a major change in your life.

We have witnessed this system working successfully for many years and this system always works, when you use it. The right kind of knowledge can be a very powerful thing in your life.

This book is about sharing knowledge that will help you look after your mind and body for the rest of your life.

Today is an age of knowledge and we have endless access to information, thanks to the internet. Everyone is educating themselves on so many topics, except for the most important areas in their lives where they do not take action. NOW is the time for you to take action.

Many people live their lives glued to the TV and reading newspapers. When they meet with their friends or colleagues at work, they normally quote what they read or saw that day on the news or something they heard someone say about the past.

When William began writing this book with Michele, he mentioned to a casual acquaintance that he had stopped watching television. Judging by the expression on her face, William could see that she was astounded. After a moment, she asked him, what he was going to do with his life if he gave up watching television. Wow, that is insane! The world has gone crazy watching TV and surfing the internet for wasted hours each day.

Funny and uplifting movies on DVD are great; however, we do recommend that you stop watching the news, crime shows, and depressing soaps. Doing this, will allow you more quality time with yourself and your loved ones. Your life will thrive.

Remember that we have free will and that we can choose which way to live our lives. People seem to live in the past or in the future, which causes them to forget about what is most important. Now!

One day, you can meet someone, the sun is shining and it is a beautiful day. What does this person say when you comment on the beautiful day? *Oh, I heard that tomorrow is going to be very bad.* Some people are unable to enjoy the beautiful weather that we have and look for bad news.

Most people have been programmed from an early age by their parents, schoolteachers and media to think in such a way.

The child will absorb these negative messages and others as if they are their own thoughts, and reinforce them repeatedly. This affects them as they grow into adulthood, especially when they have a chance to improve their life. Many times these thoughts convince you that you are not good enough or intelligent enough to progress ahead and you think to yourself, I will just stay where I am.

The same thing happens when you see a job position that you would love to have with a great salary. A great job with great pay and you do not even apply for it, because you believe that you are not smart enough. Where do you think you picked that up?

This is only one example of the many things that we have been told and now consider true.

It is the same with parents. Our parents are unaware of the damage they cause without meaning to; they always want the best for us. However when angry, many a time they use scathing words and phrases that leave indelible scars. If a child hears these often enough, they will believe it and act it out for the rest of their lives.

Many overweight people have beliefs they are not good enough or do not deserve to be happy. They feel that they do not deserve to be loved. These feelings and others, dwell within their sub-conscious mind just waiting to surface.

Have you ever noticed how some people go out of their way to destroy their relationship with their partner? Maybe you are one of them. The root cause for this self-destructive behavior can be traced back to something in a person's childhood.

You may have purchased this book because you have been searching for more than just releasing weight, you may also be searching for effective ways to make a major shift and experience real transformation in your life.

Why is it so hard to move forward? Why are other people so lucky and you are not? Why do some people have it easy and you do not?

Parts of this book will be about the do's and don'ts of foods, and the training system. In the rest of this book, we will be introducing you to the power of your mind, which will be new for some people. Once you begin reading these chapters, you will realize how much of your life has been controlled by old programs in your sub-conscious mind, that are not even your own.

We will be introducing you to affirmations, visualization, and most importantly, the Practice of Meditation.

If you can learn to practice meditation, this alone will change your life and your understanding of why your life has become stagnant. This will be a life changing experience. Imagine removing all the drama from your life.

We are aware that many people have paid out hard-earned money for ill-informed fat burning systems. Systems that they discovered were hard work, complicated and difficult to remember. Others promote the use of various types of pills. We will teach you how to do it naturally and safely.

This knowledge will enable you to look after your body for the rest of your life and teach you how your mind plays such a big part in this. We recommend food that works to burn fat and a training system that will help you achieve a flat stomach and tight, glowing skin.

There is more to this book than just assisting you to release weight. It is also about transforming your life. When you follow the steps, your life will change for the better in ways that will seem well, miraculous!

You will discover a new confidence and peace beyond all understanding and a new bounce to your step. You will not complain anymore and resentment will disappear from your consciousness. Did you know that resentment is like banging your head off a wall, and then hoping that the other person will bleed?

Some of the more popular mainstream magazines deliberately attempt to lead you astray by displaying pictures of men and women with great abdominal muscles under the heading: Get Great abs in six weeks or Build Great Abs in six weeks when actually it took more than a year to get there. These particular magazines catch the reader's attention with sensational statements because they are only interested in sales and nothing else. Certainly not the truth!

Michele was once asked if she would be in an infomercial as the AFTER for a new diet pill. Michele said, *but I have no weight to lose.* The people said, *that's okay we will be using a different model to put your face on for the before, you will be the after shot.* Michele laughed and of course said no and that they were full of bullshit and that she felt sorry for all those people who were being fooled.

We will show you what the truth is.

People feel disappointed when they see the people on the cover who looked like that in just six weeks. Well, now you know the truth, it was most likely not even them OR it took longer than six weeks to look like a Greek goddess or god.

Regrettably, if you follow the advice of most magazines and the methods that they are promoting today, you will end up doing the exact opposite of what works to create and maintain a lean body and great abs.

It will be much better if you read this book from start to finish slowly for the first time. Then on the second read, you can choose the parts you like the best and then apply them as desired. Each section can stand alone to assist you to reduce fat or you can apply them all together.

Applying them all together will do exactly what is says on the cover.

Burn fat fast, so that you will be Your Perfect Weight Looking Good and Feeling Great!

Right now, you may not feel like doing much exercise, but if you just go for a fast-paced walk and eat some of the foods we suggest, you will still reduce fat. A fast-paced walk is what your body calls fast-paced, not what other people call fast-paced.

Drink lots of water. This is very important. Say six to eight glasses a day in the first week and as your body becomes accustomed to this much water drink more miraculous water. Your body and brain will thank you. As soon as you feel thirsty, your brain is already 70% dehydrated. Your brain also requires water. Water in your tea and coffee does not count folks. PLEASE stay away from those energy drinks or energy fuel drinks. They are full of sugar and artificial sweeteners.

Many fat removal programs offer you extra bonuses that are to do with the same thing. From what we understand, they have no faith in their system so they are offering alternatives.

Let us start here.

Please understand this. As we mentioned, when you read about most diets, they show you, before and after pictures of people who were overweight. The new picture shows them as lean beautiful muscular people.

SORRY.

Diets do not build muscle and food or tablets on their own do not build muscle.

It was hard work with multiple weights in a gym and probably with a trainer. You need to work to build muscle, it does not just appear, however it is fun work, as the results make it fun!

You can build muscle without weights by training hard, but weights are the fastest way.

We have heard people say, *I do not want to look like her or him. I do not want that much muscle.*

WAKE UP! You are not going to get a body like that unless you plan to train hard with weights and machines. It takes many long hours in a gym to get that body. What are you thinking? How did you get that idea?

If you are open, we can teach you how to change your thoughts, and reprogram your own mind. We are simply guiding you so that you can throw out the garbage that is attempting to enter your life so that you can say yes to the positive and no to the negative. It is a choice. Your choice.

We will show you how to do this, but you have to want it first. If you apply the techniques here, you will start to see the change. Then you will want to change your thoughts and we will show you how.

We are asking you to look at your thoughts and to see if they are your thoughts or someone else's that you made yours.

Right now, your mind is like a piece of furniture, but instead of assembling we need to disassemble it, and clean out all the muck that you have unconsciously been holding onto.

It is your thoughts and your beliefs that keep you stuck with the extra weight.

Did you ever make a decision and say that you were going to do something Monday morning. Maybe it was to give up smoking, sweets, coffee or start something new but when Monday comes something inside of you is saying, not today maybe next week. Whom do you think just made that decision? You said you were going to do it, so why did it not happen?

We will tell you why, it is because your sub-conscious mind did not want change. It wants things to stay the same. When you try to force it to change, it fights back until you feel tired and give up.

We are here to help you with your mind, and we are not going to fight it. We are going to gently direct your sub-conscious to a new paradigm of heathy living.

If you plan on removing fat and keeping it off, then you need your mind to be ok with this. If your mind is OK with it, it will be so easy. Just make a decision right now and go for it.

Imagine going to an airport without any money and without a ticket and trying to fight your way onto a holiday flight that is fully booked. You may get on the plane, but you know that the airport police will immediately drag you off that plane.

This is the same as when you are attempting to change and remove your body fat. The mind will drag you back.

You may remove the fat, same as you getting on the flight, but you will never keep it off. Your sub-conscious mind is like the airport police. You will be stopped every time, until you give up.

You can fight it, but it will become difficult for you and make your life very unpleasant. You have to change your self-image first.

HOW IT WORKS

First, please understand why you are here. You are here to push your mind to a new limit, yes your mind, not your body. Please remember this. We will be working with your mind.

Once your mind accepts this, the body will follow. (*It is that simple*) More than likely, you have never thought about it in this light before.

Your sub-conscious mind is so simple to understand and you know this well because you have been talking and listening to it all your life. By the end of this book, you will know much more about your mind and how it affects your life.

If you had a problem before with becoming fit or removing fat, it was because you did not prepare your mind. It is like a boxer shadow boxing, there is no one there, but he is visualizing the other boxer in front of him. He is training his mind for what he wants to happen in the ring and he knows his body will follow.

The boxer does not know exactly how visualization works. He just knows through experience, that it does work. Remember that in a boxing gym there are lot of bags to punch, big ones small ones, heavy and light, yet the boxer chooses to punch an invisible person using his mind.

Today experts in many fields of sport such as running, golf, swimming, basketball and other sports are using visualizing techniques e.g. When the golfer takes the swing alongside the ball and then looks up the green as if he had hit it already. The golfer is trying to imagine the shot in his mind. This is visualization and it is part of the secret of getting what you want in life. Did you ever see a snooker player lining up the ball with his mind before he hits the ball? This is the same thing.

Your mind is a miraculous instrument, and if you understand it and work with it, you will be amazed with what you can do. Everything will become possible for you.

We will address visualization later in this book in far more detail, and make it very easy for you to understand and use.

We will put it on automatic and we will introduce you to ways of changing your mind without the fight. When you understand this, your life will get so much better

With the mind on our side, we have won. This is one of the most important lessons we can learn, to improve our lives.

If the Empire State building in New York City was filled with computers, that would still not compare to the vastness of your mind capacity. Most people do not know this, but they do not know that they do not know. Our conscious mind is so small and most of us are controlled by our sub-conscious mind. For some, this book will open up a completely new world that will make you feel like you were asleep your entire life.

This knowledge will benefit you for the rest of your life.

**If you do not go after what you want,
you will never receive it.**

**Stop thinking of what could go wrong
and start thinking of what will go right.**

GET MOVING

Before we share more about the mind and foods to avoid and what foods to eat. Let's remember to have some FUN and fun begins with moving our bodies.

Once we begin to move our bodies, we will not be able to live without movement. It will become almost as automatic as breathing. A fundamental part of every day life. Just as we take time to eat, sleep, work, love, and brush our teeth, we move our bodies.

The next few chapters you will be learning The Ten UP System™. The rest of the chapters deal with very important information about foods to eat and foods to avoid. We wish to remind you that the Ten UP System™ is way beyond regular exercise as it releases FAT FAST!

Of course, regular exercise is a critical factor in how we look, in the shape, strength (*inner and outer strength*) and suppleness of our body. It affects the tone and glow of our skin. The eyes become brighter. Exercise greatly determines how we feel and raises our energy levels, moods, mental alertness and allows our minds to have clarity. It also strengthens our bones, muscles, heart, lungs, digestive organs, blood, nerves and hormones. In addition, for those who are interested, exercise also affects our libido!

If we engage in some sort of fun exercise that raises our heart rate, just three times a week, it will not only give us longevity but it can lead to changing our thoughts to create a very fulfilling and happy life.

Very sadly, even though people know about the need to move our bodies in order to release weight, most people who have gained a lot of weight over the years, are unwilling or unable to bring themselves back to regular exercise.

This is because they have programed their minds to think it is hopeless. It is not! We have seen obese people become fitter in their later years than when they were in their twenties. It is NEVER EVER too late.

This resistance to change is not something that happens to us naturally. A lot of it is a family's influence, technological dependencies (*the internet etc.*) and sometimes the wrong friends.

When we were young most of us were VERY aware of how our bodies looked to others. We learned how our bodies felt. We just LOVED to move our bodies. It was natural and exhilarating to jump rope, skip, run, skate, and swim and truly feel alive. Somewhere along the road to adulthood things shifted and LIFE got in the way of the thrill of simply moving our bodies. When we move our bodies that movement during the day helps the body to continue to burn fat as we sleep.

We helped an unhappy young man, who had gained a lot of weight and felt hopeless. He was in a negative state of mind and did not know how to change his old thoughts and habits. He was on the internet all day at work and on the internet surfing all night. We suggested how he could change his thinking and we explained that The Ten UP System™ would be wonderful. Michele also suggested he get away from his computer and go out more. He started dance classes and not only released over 140 lbs. he also gained a girlfriend. Now he is a much happier, more fulfilled healthier human being.

Now let us cover HOW to shift your awareness and learn how to visualize. Very soon, you will actually want to move that precious body of yours.

VISUALIZATION

**I am now at my perfect weight,
looking good and feeling great.**

What a magnificent statement. We gave you that powerful affirmation song as a gift earlier in this book.

In this chapter, we are not going to speak about losing weight.

What did your mother or father tell you to do when you were just a little bit of a thing and you had lost something? Think about it. What did they teach you? They taught you to find it didn't they? Yes they did. And, we were good little kids. We learned our lessons well when we were little children. Millions of people learn that lesson so well, that they have lost and found tons in their lifetime. Literally tons of unwanted fat that has caused an untold amount of damaging frustration and anxiety, which has led to a false and distorted sense of self.

In a very short span of time, you are going to look at this system as magical.

You might be wondering what your perfect weight is. Who could tell you what your perfect weight is? Do not bother looking for a height and weight chart with this system. There isn't one. Have you ever wondered where those charts came from? Who made them? If they were accurate, they would state that if the male is six feet, then he should weigh XX. Females, who are the same height, would be at a different weight because they are females. In fact, many women who are 5'8" in height weigh more than some men who are 5'8" in height. The beautiful truth is that both of these people could be at their perfect weight.

If you want this system to work for you, then please get rid of the chart and get rid of your scales. No one knows what your perfect weight is, now hear this, read carefully, your sub-conscious knows what your perfect weight is, and we are going to give a directive to your sub-conscious mind to move your body into the vibration, which will produce your perfect weight. Now that is probably a new idea for you. However, understand it works.

Rather than lose weight, you are going to let something go that you have been holding onto. Something you do not want. Your very likely holding onto a number of things in your life that you do not want. There are many women who are holding onto men they don't want and of course, the opposite would be true.

As you become truly acquainted with this liberating concept, you will begin to see the other areas of your life where this concept can be applied. You will also see the added benefits you are going to receive because you invested in this book. You will be letting go of a number of things in your life that you do not want.

You are going to be so pleased with the future. Yes, your future is going to be exciting when you learn to live in the now and take action TODAY.

This explanation will create an awareness of how such a deceivingly simple concept can and will be truly powerful for you.

When the image, that these positive words represent in the garden of your marvelous mind, take hold, you will begin letting go of one pound after another every day. You must become emotionally involved with your new image. Put a smile on your face; bring that smile into your heart with every word. Get up and dance to the music. Let the joy in your heart be expressed through your vibrant body in action. Don't just sit passively listening, you must get involved and move!

Now please understand that the mind controls the body. We suppose you could say that you are getting involved in the abc's of perfect weight. This is not only a beginner system; it is also a graduate system all in one. Expect a miracle and you become the miracle. If you have studied the workings of the mind, you will quickly recognize the wisdom in this system.

The mind impresses the pictures of images upon the sub-conscious mind and whatever is impressed on the sub-conscious mind must be expressed in your body. Let us repeat that, must be expressed in your body. Your body is the servant of your mind.

We recommend you NEVER EVER paste pictures of fat people on your refrigerator. This simply impresses upon your mind that image. Perhaps take a person (*Not a skinny model*) who is healthy and of similar height and paste your face on THAT picture. When Michele had put on fourteen lbs. and had to release that weight fast. She worked out of course, but she also put her face on the body of Kylie Minogue, as that singer also has a petite frame, as does Michele. The new body image really helps to change the way you think and feel. Michele released those fourteen lbs. fast.

The wise men of the past were right. The picture that you hold of yourself in your heart will control your life. Your body does not have a choice. It must do what the images in your heart and in your sub-conscious mind tells it to do.

The great master artist, Michelangelo, painted a picture of the doorway to heaven. On the painting there was no doorknob because, you see, that the doorway to heaven, the doorway to a life of freedom and pure happiness, must be opened from the inside. Yes, it must be opened from within and it is time for you to open the door to a new life.

The instructions are deceivingly simple. They really are.

Write out this statement with feeling.

I willingly and lovingly release the distorted image of my beautiful true self that I have been holding. I clearly understand that all of nature abhors a vacuum. Therefore as my old distorted image of self is released and dissolves forever into the limitless ether. Spirit is filling my conscious mind with an exciting, dynamic, stunningly beautiful image of myself. My wonderful self, at my perfect weight. I am relaxed. I am not concerned with my measurements or weight. Such as the number of pounds, I weigh. I only have a beautiful picture of myself. A dynamic image of the size of my body I want to live in. This picture of me, at my perfect weight, becomes clearer every time I see it. It causes my mind and body to be filled with an emotion of sheer joy and gratitude. I know, yes I know, and I know that I know, that this image of me, this wonderful image of me, at my perfect weight, is being safely and permanently deposited in the ether. What I have just affirmed must come to pass. Love

_____

(Your Name)

41

I AM NOW AT MY PERFECT WEIGHT. LOOKING GOOD AND FEELING GREAT.

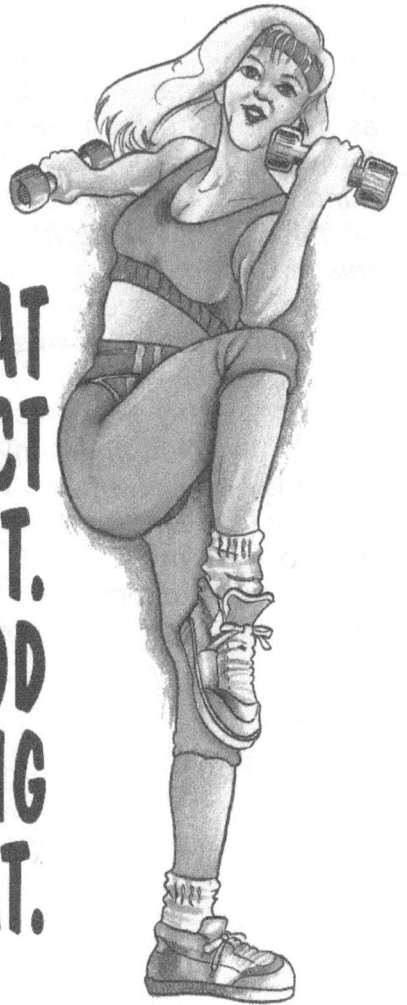

Your mind has been similar to a dirty swimming pool.

When Michele lived in Kuala Lumpur. Her apartments had a huge beautiful pool. Michele would get up early each morning and take a swim. One morning as she went for her swim she noticed the water in the pool was a very dark blue color.

A maintenance man walked over to Michele to explain what was happening, *"I'm sorry Michele you're not able to go swimming today. Someone has dumped coloring into the pool overnight. The pool will be closed for a while. We have been working on the problem all day, although no one can see the result of our efforts yet. It is quite possible that you will not see any visible change in the color of the water for a few days. There is clear, clean, unpolluted water being pumped into the pool all day long, and at the same time, the dirty, or polluted, water is being drained from the pool. It is a slow process but it is very effective. The clean clear water is weakening the colored water, but because it is happening slowly, you are not able to detect the difference with your eye. But you know if we just continue pumping clear, clean, unpolluted water in, the old polluted water, will soon be as clean and fresh as it once was, and in a few days, you can go swimming again."*

Michele shared this story with her friend Bob Proctor and he often uses this analogy at his seminars. You see our mind is like the swimming pool, at first the old self-image is still there however when we are persistent, the new image will become clear and clean, just as the swimming pool did. Be patient and persistent.

Visualizing yourself at your perfect weight will firmly plant the new idea in your heart. Now you are ready. You are at the door. You are on your way into a new world. As you open it and step forward, you will be on the right road to a bright future.

Now Let Us Begin The TEN UP SYSTEM™

THE ROPE AND CENTRIFUGAL FORCE

CENTRIFUGAL FORCE

First, we need to explain a little about physics, centrifugal forces and their importance in this training system, as this is what causes your upper body to workout

Centripetal force is a force that makes a body follow a curved path similar to a roller coaster ride.

Centrifugal force is the tendency of an object following a curved path, to fly away from the center of curvature. Centrifugal force is not a true force.

If you tie a ball onto a string of about two feet in length and start to swing the ball in a circle, the ball is said, to exert great centrifugal force on the string and can break it. The weight of the ball on the string before swinging it, can be quite light, but the faster you swing the ball the much heavier it becomes. This is called centrifugal force, as it increases the ball weight at high speed that in turn can easily break the string.

In a washing machine during the spinning cycle, clothes are forced up against the wall of the drum and the water is forced out through the small holes in the drum. Again, this is centrifugal force. Another example is a hammer thrower in sports; the faster that they can spin the further they can throw the hammer.

In order for this to work we need weight and we need speed, the Ten UP System™ rope, will give us both.

HOW TO BURN FAT FAST
WITH
THE TEN UP SYSTEM™

We are here to reduce fat so that you will become much stronger, fitter, more alert, and start to feel good about yourself.

The type of rope we will be using will be the key to getting the maximum results.

Normal skipping ropes found in sports stores will do, however you will not get the benefit of the upper bodywork from those types of ropes.

Try to avoid eating one hour before you start this system as you might get a cramp.

Later we will recommend some music that will give that extra push, as the right music can break down many barriers that can make you give up.

If you can, please buy these songs and make a play list for your workout. These particular songs have a heavy beat and they have the ability to speak to your mind. It will be like talking to your sub-conscious mind. These songs will help you remove the (*I cannot)* and replace it with (*I can*).

Many songs today may have the beat, but not the lyrics. Very few songs have positive lyrics to help you reprogram your sub-conscious mind.

The way that we are going to explain this, may seem a bit childish to some, but we are deliberately doing this, as we want everyone to understand.

You will need a skipping rope, a clock and a mirror. That is all.

Having a friend there would be a help, but only if you would like someone calling out the time for you. Turn up the music.

The special type of skipping rope that William is recommending will push your results to the maximum, as this type of rope plays a big part in the overall toning up of your upper body.

William will show you how to build this type of rope. However, if for some reason you do not want to build the rope or do not have the time, then William can make it for you. Please go to this website http://www.tenupsystem.com Let William know your height and he can customize it, just for you.

You can do this system on your own but it is much more fun doing it with a friend.

First, you need to buy a large clock with a second hand that can be seen clearly from ten feet away.

It is very important that the clock have a second hand because that is what we will be really focusing on. You can buy these types of clocks quite inexpensively.

TRAINING and AFFIRMATIONS

Later we will discuss how affirmations work in more detail, because affirmations are a very vital part of the process.

Directly in front of where you will be training, please hang or tape to the wall, signs with printed statements on them. I AM and I LOVE, are some of the most powerful words on the planet today. What you put after them is what shapes your reality and your future.

Here are some examples.

- I AM Now at my Perfect Weight Looking Good and Feeling Great.
- I AM Now so Happy and Healthy.
- I LOVE to drink lots of water every day.
- I LOVE eating foods that are healthy, fresh and filled with life-force energy.
- I AM burning fat NOW.
- I love and appreciate my body.
- Every day in every way, I AM becoming fitter and fitter and more and more toned.

When you train, look at these signs and say them with enthusiasm out loud, over and over again.

When we speak about **10 up** or **10 to go**, we mean TEN SECONDS and no more. REMEMBER THIS. Train as if your life depends on it as this is the most important time of the session and this is THE KEY.

First, we want you to feel what ten seconds is like as this is the making and breaking of the fat burning process.

Please count to ten, just like the seconds on the clock. Count them out loud now!

1, 2, 3, 4, 5, 6, 7, 8, 9, 10!

When you do this a few times, you will feel how little ten seconds truly is. There will be a time in the Ten UP System™, when you will be so focused on the ten seconds that your mind will try to play tricks by telling you that it is much longer.

It is only ten seconds. This is the key.

Count it out loud again. **1, 2, 3, 4, 5, 6, 7, 8, 9, 10.**

This is how the system works. We are going to base this on a three minute round and as you get fitter and faster you can increase the number of rounds.

However, the maximum we will ever do is twelve rounds. That is enough for the fittest of people and do not worry, whatever you are able to do **right now** is enough because, if you push your body now and three rounds is all you can do, then that is enough for you to burn fat. Three rounds was just a number we chose so don't be concerned if you do less, as that is where your body is now and we are starting from where you are, right now.

If you can build yourself up to nine rounds of a workout and include warm up time and rest periods, you will be finished in thirty-seven minutes.

Do this three times a week and the fat will fall off you.

The three-minute rounds are broken into six parts and are easy to remember. We will explain it in two ways. One with words and one with numbers to make it as easy as possible.

You will start with a warm up of two minutes or more of easy skipping similar to running on the spot.

Your Abdominals Muscles

You skip as if you are running on a field. You lift your knees high, as this is very important.

When you lift your knees, you are activating your abdominal muscles. It is actually your stomach muscles, which are lifting your legs.

When you skip this way, you will be working your lower abdominals and at the same time, burning fat from your belly.

You get two for the price of one.

Flatten your belly and tone your Abs.
How cool is that? Very cool indeed.

The first minute is twenty seconds plus ten seconds and then twenty seconds plus ten seconds once again, which gives you sixty seconds of your first minute.

You will also apply this to the second minute and the third minute of the first round.

All the rounds will be the same, 3 minutes each.

20 sec (Run) and 10 sec (Run very Fast)

20 seconds +10 seconds + 20 + 10 = 60 (1 minute)

20 seconds +10 seconds + 20 + 10 = 60 (1 minute)

20 seconds +10 seconds + 20 + 10 = 60 (1 minute)

60 Second Breaks But Keep Moving.

In between rounds, you take time out. However, do not stop. Keep moving, walking, stretching your body, anything but do not stop.

It can be good to work out in front of a mirror as you can see your skipping techniques and you can see how much better you are getting, which can be a great boost to your confidence.

If you do decide to use your own music selection then please, use a fast beat, not music with sad words, but songs with positive lyrics and a great beat.

This is part of playing with the mind.

We recommend that you purchase a small container that can spray water. In between rounds, you can spray this into your mouth, as your mouth will become dry with the intensity of the system you will be using.

In most supermarkets today, you can buy an artificial lemon and when this is emptied, you can fill it with water and use this as your spray.

Of course, we recommend you drink as much water as you can, every day.

To get the most out of this system we recommend using Williams Ten UP System™ Skipping Rope.

This system can be done running on the spot or running on the road, treadmill or even on a bike, but you will be missing the upper bodywork out. With the skipping rope, you get a total body workout.

The type of rope William is going to teach you how to easily make, works your upper body splendidly. You can start with an ordinary skipping rope or just buy one. Any sports store sells them.

The thing about skipping ropes is the heavier the better, but it must be one that can move with speed, as this is where physics come into play. They do not make this type of rope. The rope has to be heavy and fast. As mentioned, William will show you how to make the perfect rope for so little money.

It is recommended you use heavy electrical cord and William will show you with some pictures he took, how to make this with just an old brush handle, two screws, six washers and a piece of tape.

You can purchase all these items in any hardware store or online. The heavy rope, using physics, will work your upper body, arms, shoulders, chest, and upper back.

Here is how it works.

You start your skipping at the top of the minute.

You skip for the first twenty seconds as if you are running lifting your knees at a jogging pace.

Lifting your knees is very important.

After the twenty seconds, you run as fast as you can for (ten seconds.)

Do this for the three minutes. If you start doing this in a group, you would have one person watching the clock and shouting out the time.

The way we would do it would be. Skip for twenty seconds. Shout then. (Ten UP) you give it everything like you are running for your life. After the ten seconds is up you shout (ease off) and go back to the jogging pace again for twenty seconds.

You work like this for three minutes. Then you shout (time) and you walk around for fifty seconds and then for the ten seconds to the top of the minute you get ready to start your next three minute round.

Next, you do the same as the first round and so on.

This system has a powerful ability to charge up your metabolism to a new rate where your body will need extra fuel, and your fat will be used as that extra fuel.

What is going to happen next?

This interval training will set your body on a new mode, where it will push itself to an area of hard work for ten seconds. These ten seconds will take your body to a new level. Your body will then adjust to stay at that level. Remember this is only ten seconds.

When you push your body to a new level, your heart, which is a muscle, will be taken out of its comfort zone and will have to pump more blood throughout the body to get back to its normal rate. Now your body and metabolism will start to function at a much higher rate.

It is at this rate that your body will start to burn fat like never before; your metabolism will carry on burning the fat even when you are finished training. You will have started or triggered an afterburner effect and your body will still be burning calories for hours after you have stopped skipping. (*Even while you are sleeping...Awesome!*) After this, drink lots of water. Your body will need water.

The first thing you will notice is that you sweat a lot in the session and right after you finish your session. If you get up on scales, you *will* notice a weight drop.

One night, one person called Kieran dropped thirteen pounds, as he was getting ready for a weigh-in for the national championships, and after that, he went to the Olympics and came home with an Olympic medal.

This is not the weight drop we are looking for.

Most of the weight that is released is simply water that is retained under the skin. This will come back very quickly when you eat and drink again. This is a false weight drop, and this is one of the reasons why, we stay away from the scales.

What we are looking for is the fat burning process to begin and to carry on working even for hours after we have stopped the session.

You will be setting your metabolism on over drive, which will just keep burning the fat.

The first thing you will notice is your skin will start to tighten up, as this is the first sign. Stay away from scales, as they will only confuse you. You will be burning fat and at the same time, you will be building lean muscle to support your progress. A fact, muscle weighs more that fat. This type of muscle will not stand out in your body, but you will feel it in the new strength and the new energy you experience.

You will be setting your metabolism to over drive, which will just keep burning the fat.

Remember to drink lots of water.

THE FIVE-MINUTE SYSTEM

(ONLY IF YOU ARE FIT)

Remember to drink lots of water.

Make sure that you have read the Ten UP System™ first as this will explain the correct way to skip.

For this system, you will really need the music that we recommend.

The second system is one that you may not believe can work so amazingly, that is until you experience it for yourself. Then you will believe how magically this system works.

VERY IMPORTANT

- Do the five-minute system for only one round, as one round is enough.

- One round consists of five minutes. Yes just Five Minutes. That is it.

- This is a stand-alone system.

- This is the five-minute system.

- You do the same as the 10 seconds but you change it to 20 seconds.

Here is how it goes...

Twenty seconds you run and then the next 20 seconds you run at your top speed. Yes, you run all out. Twenty seconds you run and then twenty seconds at your fastest speed.

Run   **Fast**   **Run**

20 seconds + 20 seconds + 20 seconds = 1 minute

Fast   **Run**   **Fast**

20 seconds + 20 seconds + 20 seconds = 2 minutes

Run   **Fast**   **Run**

20 seconds + 20 seconds + 20 seconds = 3 minutes

Fast   **Run**   **Fast**

20 seconds + 20 seconds + 20 seconds = 4 minutes

Run   **Fast**   **Run**

20 seconds + 20 seconds + 20 seconds = 5 minutes

This enough for the fittest of people. This will send your metabolism into overdrive like never before.

Again, drink lots of water after this.

The Five-Minute System is not as easy, however it is simple and the result will speak for itself. To complete the five-minute system you must remain in the moment and please stay focused. It would be best to have some support with some friends or a skipping partner to encourage you, and listen to music with a fast beat. Music with a fast beat really helps.

RECOMMENDED MUSIC FOR
THE TEN UP SYSTEM™

William has trained for many years with this system, and he knows how helpful the right songs with the right beat can be when you are going for it!

William always searches for songs that have a beat that would work in conjunction with the rhythm of the speed of the rope and his body. He found that some songs were uplifting and helped him to work faster and longer. The songs also helped him have fun with his workouts.

Remember when we spoke about putting garbage into your sub-conscious mind and then expecting different results in your life. This segment is about clearing your mind of negativity. The lyrics of a song affect the left hemisphere of our brain and the music and melody affects the right hemisphere of our brain. Therefore, we have a whole brain experience while we are working out.

This is how Michele created her MusiVation™ songs. She was in a near fatal car accident and as a singer songwriter she was guided to begin retraining her mind to help heal her body. It really works! Her body healed very quickly. Her doctors were amazed at the results.

The only person you should be better than today, is the person you were yesterday.

Finding your enthusiasm to exercise is as simple as listening to one song that you have conditioned yourself to associate with energy and positivity. When Michele begins her workout she first puts on Pharrell Williams song HAPPY. You can find your own song. Select a song with an uplifting message that makes you want to move. The goal here is to program your mind to know that when you hear that song, you are going to work out. What you are doing is creating a connection between the song and your enthusiasm to work out. Eventually you will reach a point at which hearing the song accelerates your heart rate and breathing. This only takes one song, however cueing up four more energizing songs is great to keep your motivation on high.

The benefits of music improves your endurance, strength, and power while making you feel as if you are not working hard. Music also drowns out your thinking so that you will not hear that naughty little voice that tells you to quit.

The right playlist can also assist you form and maintain your new workout routine. If you get tired of a song delete it and find another song that keeps you uplifted. Do not put your playlist on shuffle. Make sure you have carefully chosen the songs that keep you motivated. We recommend you buy these songs and put them on a play list for when you are training.

These songs make you feel good. All the way through your training time, you will be receiving positive programing of your choice, into your sub-conscious mind. Remember what we said about the blue dye in your swimming pool earlier. These songs are like clean fresh water that is pouring new positive thoughts into the swimming pool of your mind. Experiment with working out with these positive songs and see the results.

Suggested Songs

- **Starlight,** by Matt Cardle from the movie Fast girls
- **Good Feeling,** by Flo Riha
- **Happy,** by Pharrell Williams
- **Make you Believe,** by Lucy Hale
- **Bless myself,** by Lucy Hale
- **I Got You** (I Feel Good) by James Brown
- **Reach Me,** by Michele Blood
- **Synergy,** By Michele Blood & Bob Proctor
- **Persistence,** by Michele Blood and Bob Proctor
- **Perfect Weight,** By Michele Blood & Bob Proctor
- **I Am Energy,** by Michele Blood
- **Shake Your Booty,** By K.C. & The Sunshine Band
- **The Monster,** by Eminem & Rihanna
- **Boomerang,** by Nicole Scherzinger
- **One In Million,** by Swiss, Music Kidz
- **Wide Awake,** by Katy Perry
- **Fire Work,** by Katy Perry
- **Guide me God,** by Ghostland Featuring Natacha Atlas & Sinéad O'Connor
- **Praise You** (Radio Edit), by Fatboy Slim
- **Jump Around,** by House Of Pain
- **Hey Ya,** by Outcast
- **One Day,** by Charice
- **You Can`t Touch This,** by M.C. Hammer
- **Eye of the Tiger,** by Survivor

SUMMING UP,
THE TEN UP SYSTEM™

- You will have a large mirror.

- You will also have built or bought a skipping rope with electric cable that can move fast.

- A large clock that will sit under or over the mirror, or simply on a wall in front of you where the second hand is clearly visible.

- Around the mirror or the clock, you will have six A4 paper sheets with, I AM and I LOVE statements written on them.

- You will have downloaded the songs and made a play list of the music that we have recommended for you to use, when you are skipping. Of course, you may also find other music that has great lyrics and a great beat. Experiment and have fun.

- These songs make it so much easier for you than sad or mediocre music.

- If you are using an MP3 player or an IPod, make sure that you have earphones that will not fall off or move around.

HOW TO MAKE THE TEN UP SYSTEM™ SKIPPING ROPE

The rope that we would normally use does not exist for sale anywhere. William built all of the skipping ropes.

What makes this rope different to the other ropes available, is its weight, because the weight forces your upper body to move at higher speed and hence creates upper body toning and strength.

It is a much heavier rope than the normal rope that people are using today and because of this, when you are doing the The Ten UP System™ the rope becomes much heavier in your hands because of the centrifugal force. This is when your upper body has to start working to keep up with the flow of the rope.

At the start it will feel a little bit awkward, but give it a week and you will be skipping with ease. Give it two weeks and you will be skipping as if it was something you did all your life.

You will be doing it in no time, you will even find ways of entertaining yourself with the skipping rope, doing double jumps, cross overs where you cross your hands but never stop skipping. It can be great fun.

Ok, this is how it will go.

You need to purchase a brush handle. One that is thin enough for your hand to fit around it comfortably. They are normally about four feet in length. We will be using all of this stick, as what we have cut off we need to make our handles for the skipping rope. The rest of the handle, which is left over, we will be using for our stomach/abs work out. All of these exercises will be done standing up. This is not part of the work out system, but it is good for you to know exercises that work and will make your stomach strong, which then supports your lower back. So many people have problems with their lower back. We will speak about your lower back later on in the book.

You will need two screws, six washers, a roll of tape and a length of wire, which are all available in any hardware store. The wire should have three strands inside of it and this wire is called single-phase wire. The length will be approximately two feet higher than yourself, as this is the easiest way to measure it for your height.

Once you have these, you are ready to build your rope.

THE ROPE

Read first before you start so that you will understand what to purchase.

(1) You hold the stick in your hand at one end. Just slightly longer than your hand and you mark it with a pen. You do the same at the other end.

(2) Now, you cut where you have marked the stick.

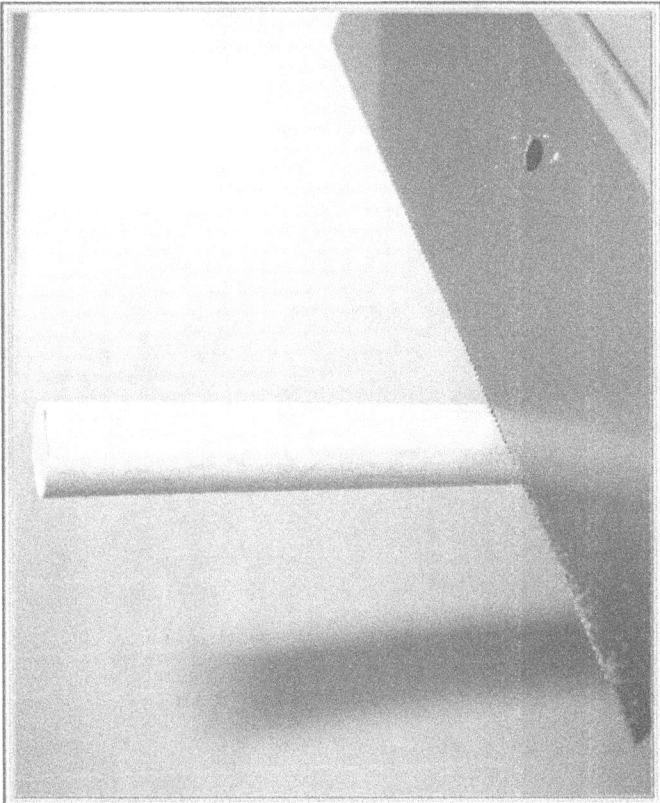

(3) Now, you have two handles that fit comfortably in your hands. You can put the rest of the stick away for now.

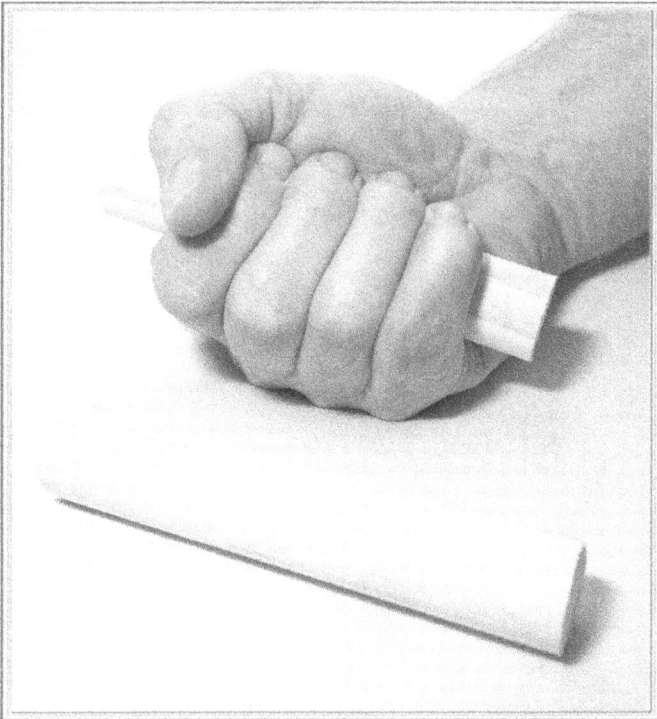

(4) Next, mark the center of the handles at one end.

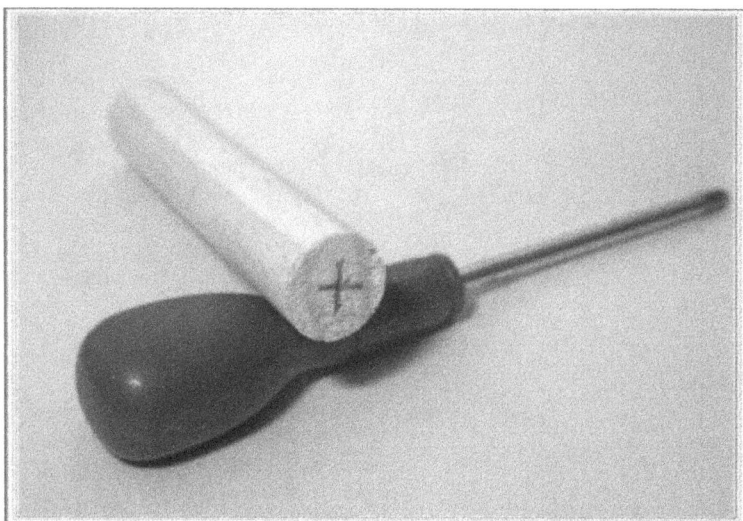

(5) Next, drill a small hole in this marked spot.

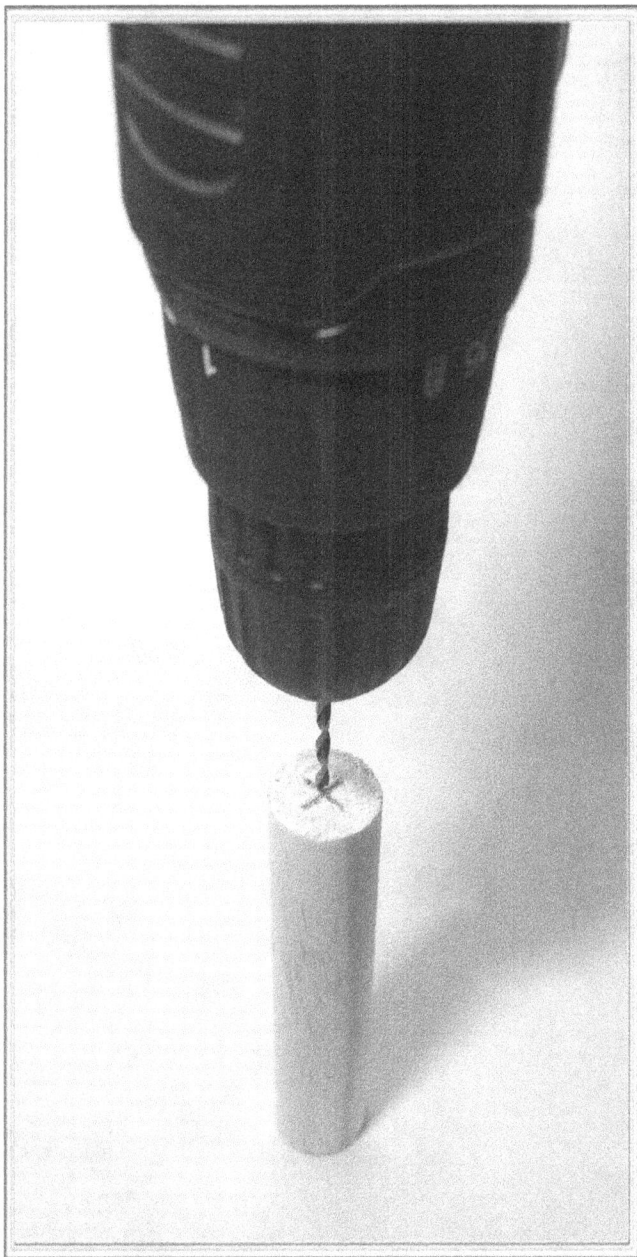

6) You will need two screws, two small washers and four large washers.

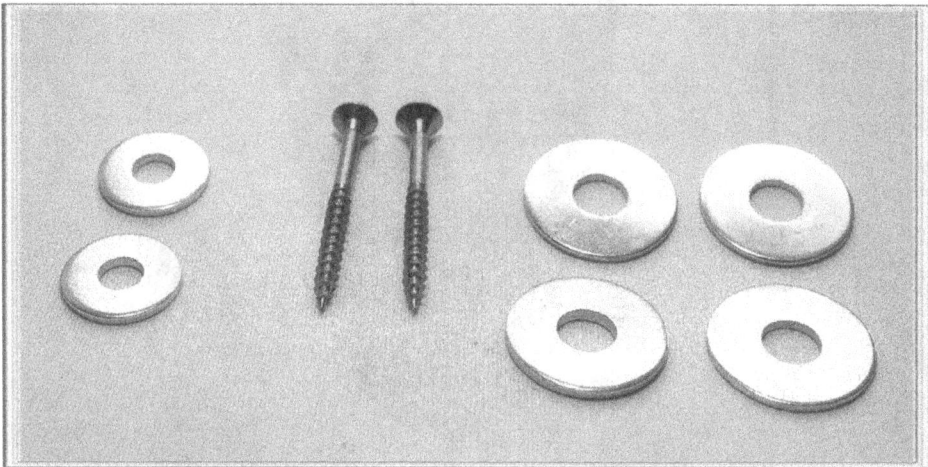

(7) You put your three washers through the screw.

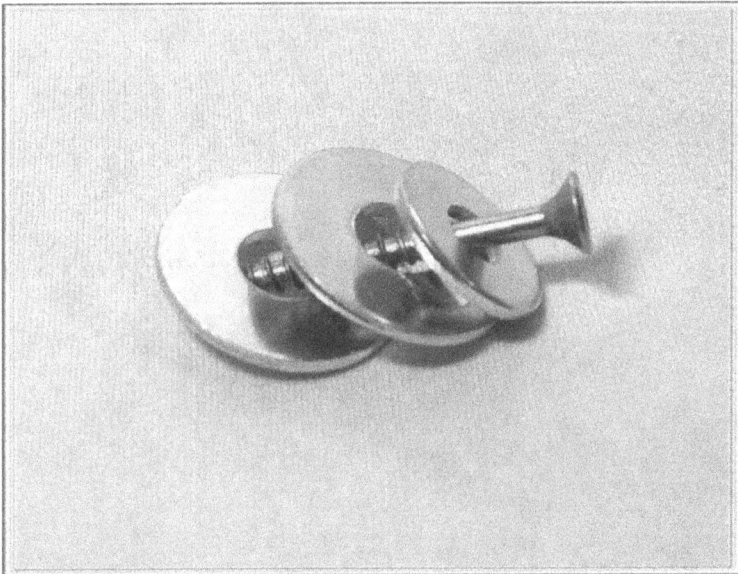

(8) Now, you screw in the screw to the center hole. Do this about half way, because you will require enough space for the rope to move freely on the screw.

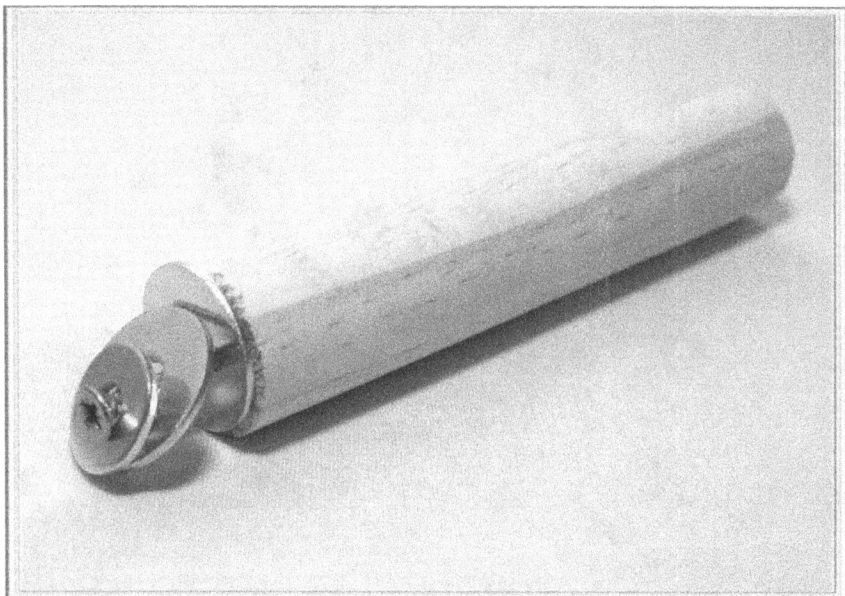

(9) Take the rope and hold it in your two hands. Now stand on the rope with your two feet. Put your hands by the side of your hips where your pockets would be. Where the rope is coming out the back of your hand, is where you cut it. Leave an extra two inches so that you can cut some off later, just in case you have made a mistake.

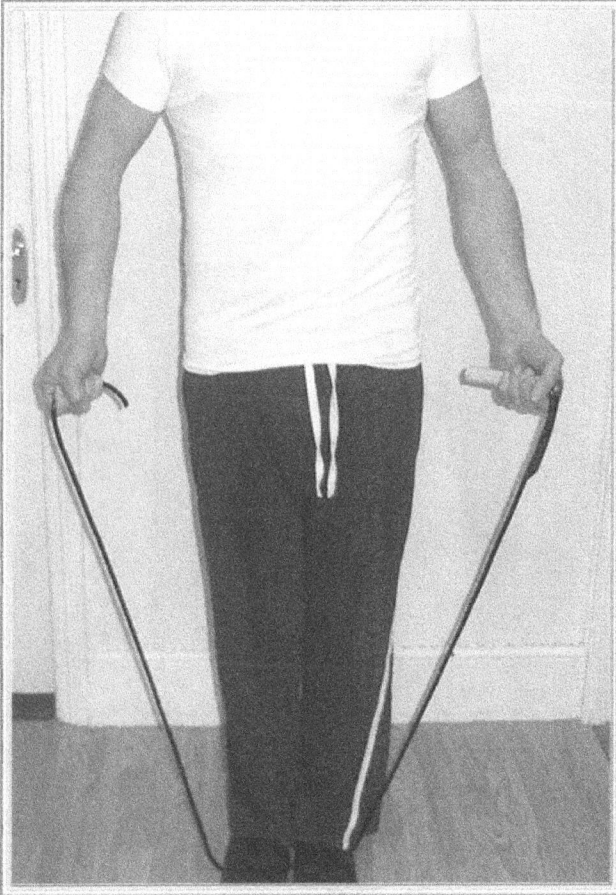

(10) Take one end of the rope and bend it over the screw in between the washers.

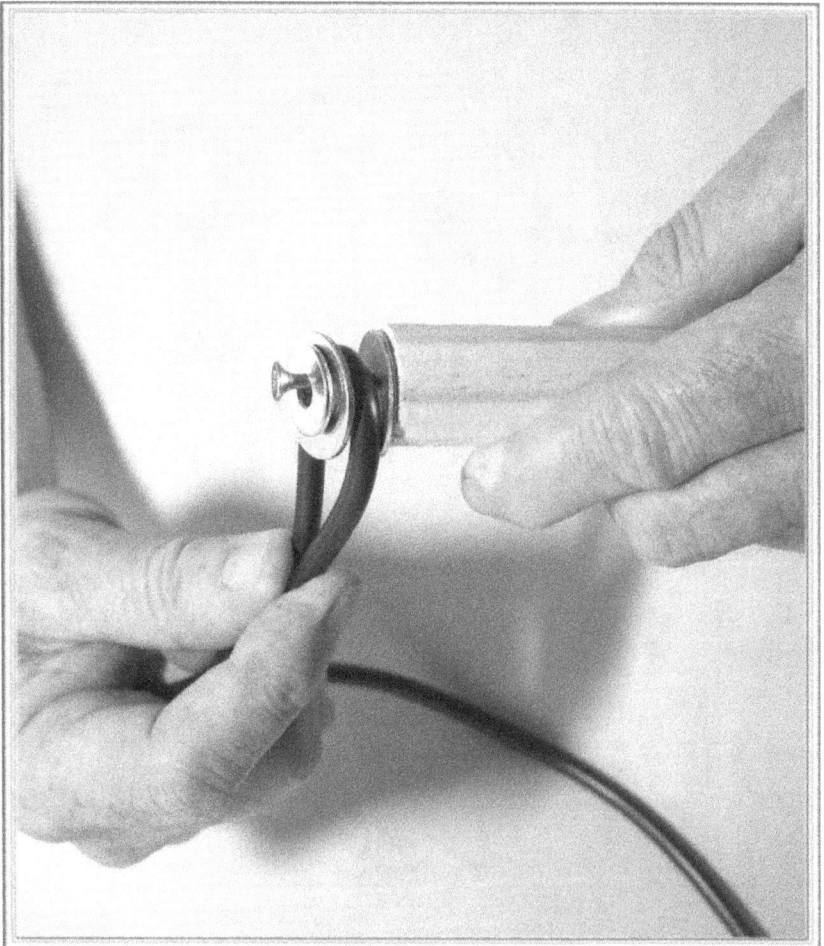

(11) Now, use the tape and tape the end of the rope onto the other part. Do one side first.

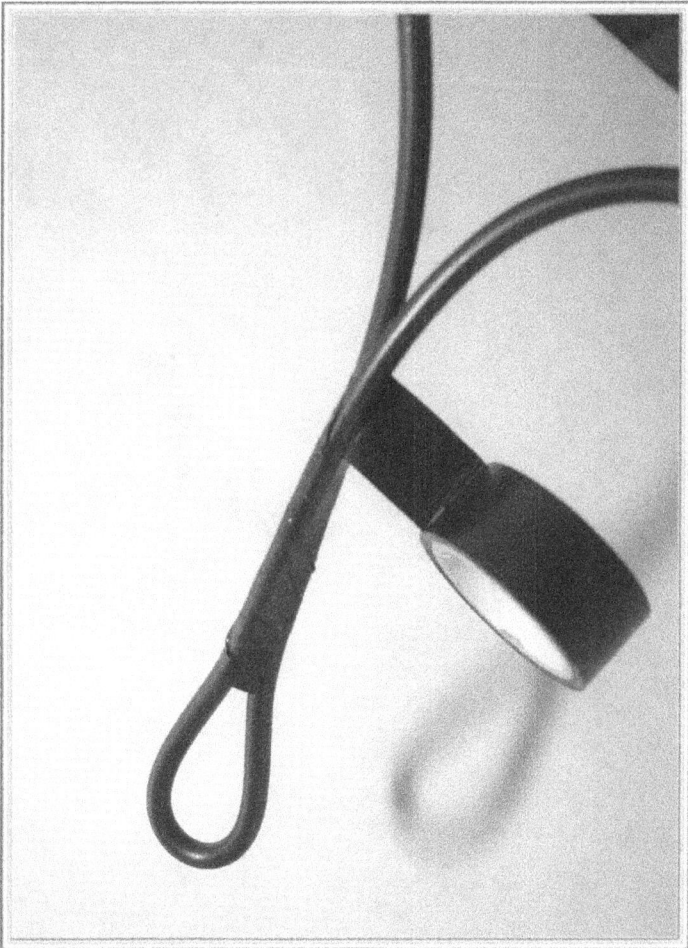

(12) Next, tape it over completely.

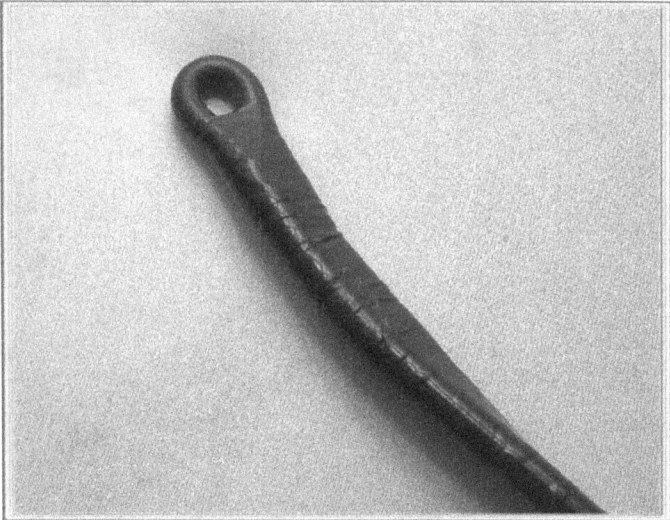

(13) This is how it will look.

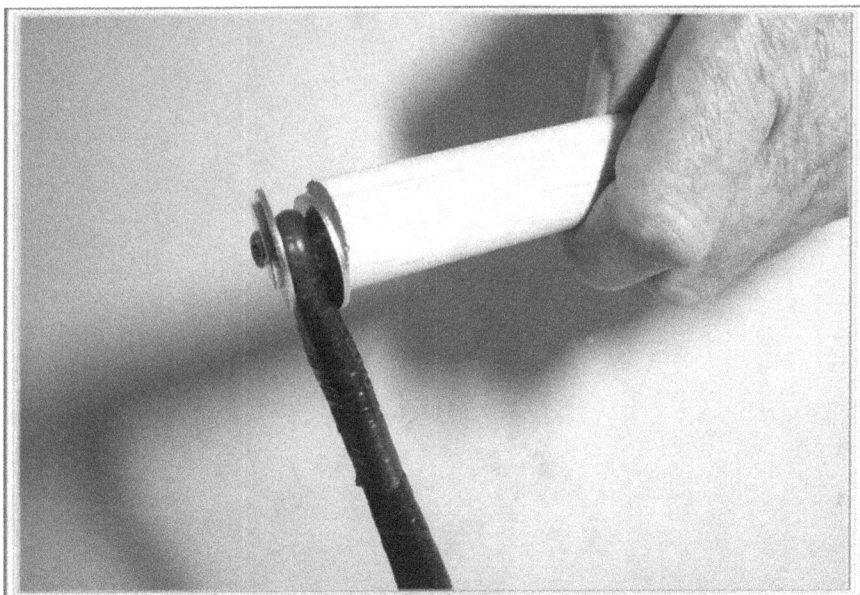

(14) Now, take the handle with the finished side in your hand and put the rope under your feet again. Hands by your hips. Cut the rope where it is coming out of the back of your hand.

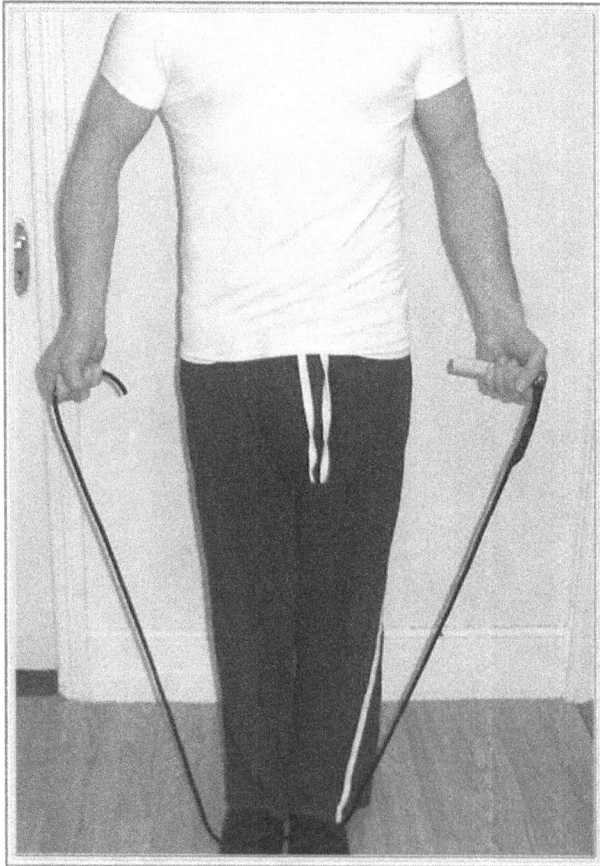

(15) Repeat step ten and eleven again on the other side.

(16) Check if the rope is the right size by keeping your hands close to your hips. Now swing the rope over your head. Please remember your hands should stay close to your body. This is quite important, as with centrifugal force the rope will be heavier with the more speed you build up.

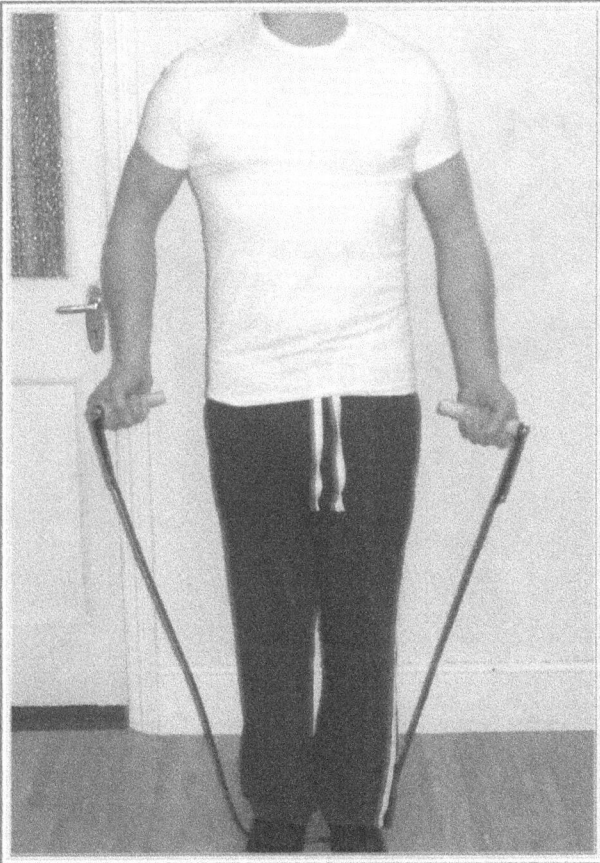

(17) Voilà! Finished product.

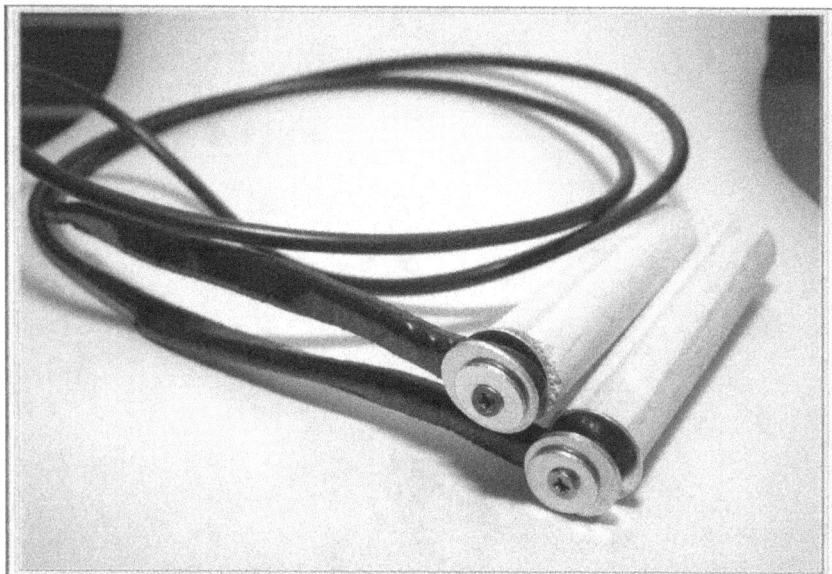

Now we can start

It would be a great help, if you could ask for motivation from a friend, as this will keep you on track in the beginning of your training.

**Every accomplishment starts with
the decision to begin.**

**If you have failed before with your
plan a, b, and c, and you are ready to quit,
please don't worry, because there are another
23 letters in the alphabet.**

REMEMBER, YOU CAN DO IT!

A very important reminder that water is very important on the fat removal list; because the more you drink the more fat will be washed out as toxins.

Water is life force energy and without it, you cannot survive.

When you awake in the morning, we recommend that you drink one eight oz. glass of water. If you can drink two x eight oz. glasses even better. After a week of drinking water, first thing every morning you will feel fantastic. Drink water before you do anything else, and continue to drink the same quantity every hour.

This will cut back drastically on your hunger and help flush out the bad toxins from your body.

This is a free and healthy way to detox your body. If you have to purchase bottled water, simply purchase a water purify for your kitchen tap and you will be free to drink as much water as you desire. You will find that the more water you drink during the day, the less hungry you will become and you will have less cravings for junk or processed food. Processed foods have additives to make you crave more junk.

Just by doing this one simple thing you will start decreasing fat straight away and reducing your body size.

It is simple, right.

Yes it is. Water, water and more water. The more water you drink, the more fat is released and you will discover your true healthy body.

YOU CAN DO IT!

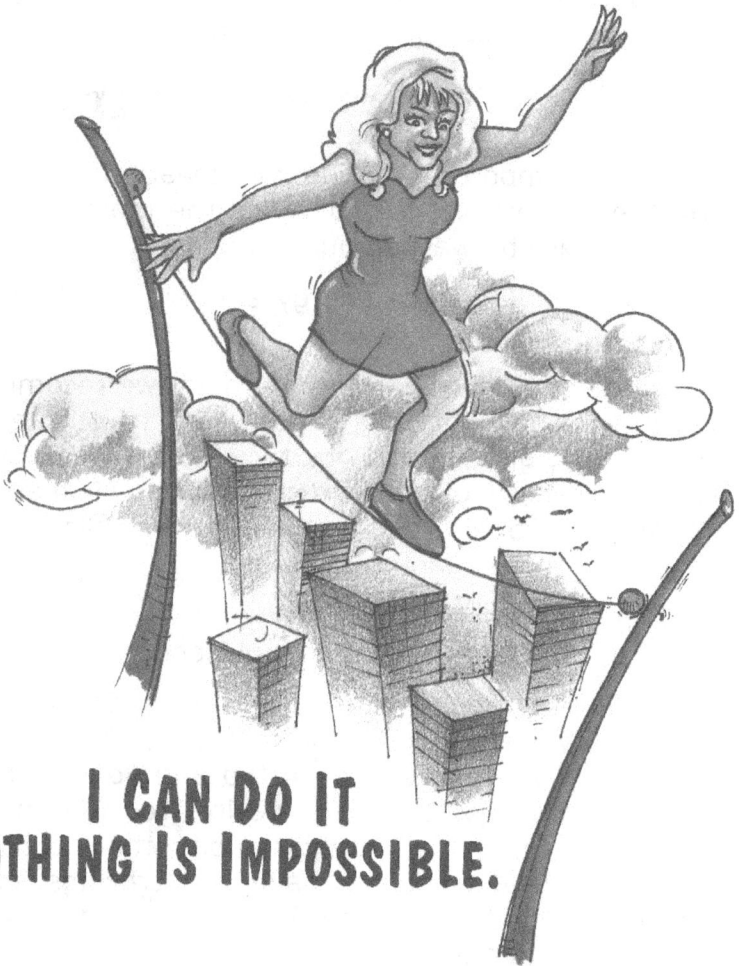

I CAN DO IT
NOTHING IS IMPOSSIBLE.

WHO IS IN CHARGE?
THE KEY TO YOUR SUCCESS

We spoke earlier about the desire to start something new e.g., a diet on a Monday morning however when the day arrives, a battle may begin. Beware of that little voice in your head that will say things like, I cannot do it, it is too hard, and I do not have the time.

Remember slim and toned *feels* better than those fatty foods and candy taste.

In the book User Illusion: Cutting Consciousness Down to size by Danish science journalist, Tor Norretrande, he cites research, based on several experiments that consciousness is limited to processing about sixteen bits of information per second, compared to the sub-conscious mind, which is processing eleven million bits of information per second.

He cites research that shows how the intellect is only conscious of fifteen to twenty bits of information per second out of millions taking place below its awareness.

If it is not our intellect, then the question is.

WHO IS REALLY IN CHARGE?

If you were not aware of what is holding you back in life, and do not learn from this, you will always struggle in life.

Your sub-conscious mind is like a herd of elephants, and your conscious mind is like a fly. They have to move together. If the herd of elephants decides to go west and the fly wants to go east, which direction do you think they will go?

From this moment on, be aware of this when you are making a decision. See, feel and notice what is happening inside of you and not outside.

At the start of this book, we mentioned that we would work on bringing your mind on board and your body will follow.

CONSCIOUS
AND
SUB-CONSCIOUS ALIGNMENT

Diet alone — or exercise alone — will not cut it.

The path to long-term, sustainable weight loss is a **healthy diet and regular exercise.** Those who elect to try one without the other are making the whole process of releasing weight that more difficult. Good eating habits, exercise, and consistency are the keys. Instead of trying to cut five hundred calories a day from your diet, it is much simpler to cut just two hundred or three hundred, and make up the rest of the calorie deficit by working out. Don't discount resistance training either. The muscle tissue you will develop will allow your body to burn calories much more efficiently, even while at rest.

If your Conscious mind wants to do one thing and your Sub-conscious mind wants something else (*counter-intention*) it will be very challenging to create what you truly want in life.

You have to resonate on all levels with what you truly wish to accomplish. You may have seen people who go on strict diets and reduce their body size while battling all of the time, and then they put the weight back on again.

The reason for this is their conscious and sub-conscious were not working together. Both of them had counter intentions and were out of alignment.

Have you heard of people winning the lottery, and losing it all in three years? The winner's sub-conscious mind regulated back to what it had habitually resonated with and it did not resonate with that much money.

It is like an air conditioner. You set it for say seventy degrees. It will stop, start, and always return to seventy degrees. This is how our mind works when we have *not* fed it the new self-image of you at your Perfect Weight Looking Good and FEELING Great!

BELIEVE YOU CAN, AND YOU CAN!

WHAT FOODS TO EAT

DRINK LOTS OF WATER.

The formula for fat release is not complicated. All you have to do is follow these easy steps and Never Give Up!

Avoid diet foods altogether and eat natural foods. Natural unprocessed foods taste so good and our body just loves them. Natural foods are the very best for fat reduction. Most of us have been misinformed and made to believe that we need some kind of processed manufactured food to release weight.

No diets, no calorie counting and no weight checks here, just fat reduction and tighter skin that simply glows.

Please do not weigh yourself. Get off those scales. You will reduce your weight, but that is not what to focus on.

Our focus is to be happy, reduce our body size and to feel great while we are becoming our PERFECT WEIGHT!

If you must weigh yourself, please experiment. Do not weigh yourself for say thirty days, while continuing to eat only natural foods. Some people's bodies have stored a lot of fat. Eating these natural foods will start to reverse this, as your body will stop storing and start burning this fat for energy. This takes time, but you will witness the difference in your body, as it will become leaner, stronger and healthier.

A simple way to check your fat reduction is to try on your clothes and see how they fit. Check once every four weeks. Then you will notice a big difference.

By making better food choices, you can improve your health and your life. When your health is good, life feels so much better.

Look after your precious body as you only have one in this lifetime.

STRESS

STRESS can be a major factor in not being able to reduce fat. We will give you some stress buster tips soon and address this further.

We will teach you how to erase stress from your everyday life and how to control your mind chatter with the practice of meditation. This is life changing. When you find your mind wandering into the past or worrying about things that have not yet happened this is a strong indication that your mind is in control, instead of you being in control of your mind. Your mind is like a cluttered house and it is very hard to move around in a cluttered house. You need to de-clutter your mind. De-cluttering your mind with the practice of meditation and the tool of mindfulness to take back control of your life.

So let us run through some of the foods that will help you in releasing fat.

If you can stop eating for four hours before you go to sleep, you will see great results.

It is vital that you cut out all fried food. If you absolutely must fry, do it at a low heat with ghee butter, or extra virgin olive oil. Just simmer on low rather that fry with too much heat because overheating destroys all those natural fat burning minerals and vitamins.

If you plan to make your own ghee, use unsalted butter.

Please do not use a microwave oven, as it destroys most of the nutrition from the food.

Another misconception is that "Fat makes you Fat". WRONG. Some fats will actually help you to reduce bodyweight because there are good and bad fats. Why this is a secret, we do not know.

The right kind of fat can help your metabolism release unwanted fat. Your body needs all three of the Macronutrients: protein, fat and carbohydrates. Our bodies need their nutrients, vitamins, and minerals.

Right now, we are just going to keep this simple and tell you the best foods to eat in order to stop storing fat. We will do this without going into too much detail of how and why this works.

When the majority of us buy a mobile/cell phone, we have no idea how it works and are solely interested in the fact that it does work. However, if you are interested in learning how good and bad fats work, then you can research the information through the internet.

There are good fats and bad fats, good carbohydrates and bad carbohydrates, just as there is good cholesterol and bad cholesterol.

Everyone talks about the bad and they never mention the good. Why is that do you think?

If you are interested perhaps, you can google the foods that we are going to introduce. Some are good for cholesterol, some for diabetes and some lower your blood pressure and fat.

If you do choose to check these foods out PLEASE check websites that are *not* trying to sell you something, as they will be honest. Other sites are interested in marketing their products and are not interested if you release fat. They are solely interested in making money. Please do not visit sites where they ask the public for their opinions, as most of the people on these sites are there because they have nothing better to do. Their answers and opinions are not based on science or fact.

Most of these sites are trying to sell you their products for diets, weight and fat reduction. Some have doctors and nutritionists strengthening their claims. Remember, doctors, nutritionists and other health specialists are just people.

Just because they received a degree to hang on the wall, does not make them a saint. They want to make easy money. Please remember the doctors who asked Michele to be in their infomercial and asked her to lie and say she had lost weight through their product. Michele could not believe that was even legal and she wondered how they could get away with such deceit. However, these people do this all the time. Do not be fooled. You are an intelligent person and you make up your own mind.

Please stay away from these sites and their claims about the benefits of their new so-called "secret" diets.

Now let us begin with some foods that are great for your body and then the foods you should stay away from in order to help you reduce your fat storing.

LATEST STUDY

ON

PROCESSED FOOD

A study of half a million people across Europe suggests that a daily diet that includes meat pies, sausages, bacon and ready meals is linked to an increased risk of dying young.

The researchers, writing in the journal "BMC Medicine", stated that chemicals used to preserve meat might damage health.

Meat consumption and mortality - results from the European Prospective Investigation into Cancer and Nutrition, Published March 7th, 2013

This major study, based on findings in 10 European countries, highlights the links between, red processed meats, heart disease and cancer. Well, you are intelligent.

Do we hear a DUH? Of course, you know that.

Findings suggest that people who eat more than 160g of these products in a day (*the equivalent of about three sausages*), have a much greater chance of dying prematurely.

Highly processed meat consumption led to a 72% increased risk of dying from heart disease, and an 11% increased risk of dying from cancer.

It also showed that people who ate processed meat were also more likely to be OBESE. i.e. - fat stored in your body, and more likely to participate in other behaviors known to damage their health.

They are talking about processed meat here and NOT red meat. In fact, they say that a little red meat does no harm.

Red meat can be enjoyed as part of a healthy, balanced diet. Opting for leaner cuts and using healthy cooking methods, such as grilling, will help keep your heart healthy.

This study was carried out over a period 12.7 years.

Professor Sabine Rohrmann from the University of Switzerland, who led the study, said that risks of dying younger from cancer and cardiovascular disease increased with the amount of processed meat eaten.

It was pointed out, that red meat also contains potentially harmful saturated fat and cholesterol. However, these were present at much higher levels in processed meat products as well as preservatives and colorants linked to cancer.

The authors pointed out that red meat contains essential nutrients and minerals that might be missing from a vegetarian diet.

However, the people who ate the most processed meat also tended to eat less fruit and vegetables.

Their Conclusions.

The results of their analyses suggest that men and women with a high consumption of processed meat are at an increased risk of early death, in particular due to cardiovascular diseases but also to cancer. Reducing the amount of processed meat consumed to less than 20g a day, would prevent more than 3% of all deaths related to cardiovascular disease and cancer.

As processed meat consumption is a modifiable risk factor, health promotion activities must include specific advice on lowering processed meat consumption.

If you want to read some reports, here are the links:

http://www.biomedcentral.com/1741-7015/11/63/abstract

http://www.biomedcentral.com/content/pdf/1741-7015-11-63.pdf

The Foods

The secret to reducing fat without going hungry is to gain knowledge and then make the right food choices. You need to choose foods that are healthy and not the foods that your body cannot process and will only end up storing as some form of fat.

Here are some of the foods that will help you *reduce fat.* There are others but these are good for a start.

Some you will love.

We will start with the big guns first.

Eggs are great for reducing fat, but if you have high cholesterol eat only the white of the eggs.

Grilled or baked fish, free-range chicken, turkey or lean organic steak. All nuts must be raw and unsalted. If you boil vegetables, you can drink the water, as it now holds all the vitamins and minerals from the vegetables and is quite tasty. Steaming your vegetables is much better. Green and Oolong teas consists of caffeine, so if you have high blood pressure, you need to watch how much you drink.

Drink lots of water. Your body and brain needs water. Aim for eventually five liters per day and then as your body becomes accustomed begin drinking one gallon per day. This one action will give you fast results.

FOODS TO EAT

Fruit & Vegetables

Apples
Artichokes
Asparagus
Beets
Blackberries
Blueberries
Bok Choy
Broccoli
Brussell Sprouts
Cabbage
Carrots
Cauliflower
Celery
Chicory
Chilies
Cucumber
Eggplant
Fennel
Garlic
Green Beans
Kale
Leeks
Lettuce
Mushrooms
Onions
Parsnip
Peppers
Radish
Rhubarb
Runner Beans
Scallions
Spinach
Sprouts
Sweet potato only
Turnips
Watermelon
Zucchini

Meats/Protein

Free range Turkey
Free Range Chicken
Halibut
Lean Steak
Mackerel
Most fish wild is preferred
Salmon
Sardines
Tuna
Free-range eggs

Liquids & Spices

Cinnamon
Cocoa
Coriander
Dark chocolate
Ginger root
Ginseng
Green tea
Humus
Mustard
Nutmeg
Oolong tea
Raw cacao powder
Saffron
Water

FOODS TO EAT (Continued)

Nuts/Fruits

Almonds
Avocado
Chestnuts
Citrus Fruits
Cranberries
Elderberries
Flax Seed
Grapefruit
Kiwi
Mango
Unsalted raw nuts
Peaches
Pears
Pecans
Prunes
Pumpkins
Raisins
Raspberries
Raw Cashew nuts
Rhubarb
Strawberries
Tangerines
Tomato
Walnuts
Wolfberries/goji berries

Oils/Milks/Flours

Almond flour
Almond oil
Avocado oil
Coconut flour
Coconut milk
Coconut oil
Extra virgin olive oil
Omega 3 pure fish oil
Organic Greek yogurt

If you have to eat cereals in the morning, then eat Oatmeal/rolled oats with no extras. Always read the back of the pack.

Stay away from processed food. A good rule of thumb is if you cannot read or pronounce the ingredients then do not eat it.

To add taste to your meals you can add:

Apple cider vinegar
Balsamic vinegar
Basil
Bay leaf
Black pepper
Cayenne pepper
Chives
Cinnamon
Cloves
Coriander
Crushed dried chili flakes
Extra Virgin Olive Oil
Honey
Lemon
Malt vinegar
Mint
Mustard
Paprika
Parsley
Real butter
Rosemary
Saffron
Sage
Thyme
Vanilla bean

A great meal taster is to add mustard and honey. As you can see, there are many types of foods to choose.

You can use stevia as a sweetener, *(it is not recommended to use it if you are trying to become pregnant)*

Nearly all of the above herbs and spices can be found in most supermarkets.

These are just a few examples of the foods that will help you reduce fat, as there are many others.

Our website will support and offer you many recipes that you will love and more foods that you can eat.

Some people recommend skipping breakfast, but it is *after* breakfast that you need your strength and energy for the rest of the day.

It is better to go without food in the evening than miss your breakfast. As the words imply you are breaking your fast. Please do not go hungry. Drink some water and eat some raw organic almonds in the evening to curb appetite. Actually eating a few almonds during the day is also good for you and assists in taking away hunger pangs.

WHAT NOT TO EAT

Try not to come to this page too often, and just focus on the foods that are good for you.

SUGAR, SUGAR, SUGAR, SUGAR, SUGAR. This is the number one enemy of your body. Next, Starch, as in flour, bread, even whole meal bread. These starches have added to that belly fat, that you have found so difficult to reduce. Breakfast cereals are full of sugar. Reduce your salt intake, as there is a lot of salt in most foods already. Do not cook with lard or fats.

MYTH BUSTER about ORANGE JUICE

Years ago, companies advertised their products in the following manner: Our product contains 10% real orange juice! Nowadays they still unashamedly write orange juice on the label. Those of us who may wish to read the contents discover that it is not possible unless we are the owners of a magnifying glass or mini microscope.

Concentrated orange juice, first thing in the morning adds too much sugar to your bloodstream. It will make you crave sweets and for some will make their stomachs too acidic. We repeat, DO NOT drink concentrated orange juice. You are much better off eating a real orange and getting all that great fiber. What is wonderful for your system first thing is some lemon juice with a large glass of water. Fruit juice and almost all the sodas drinks are full of sugar, even the ones where diet appears on them.

Read the labels and see what is really in the drink. You probably will not understand half of it and if that is the case best to avoid it all together

Avoid all processed foods.

Avoid tinned berries or any tinned fruits with processed sugar or syrup. Avoid Energy drinks and all types of fuel drinks. Anything in a tin really.

Stay away from tinned food. There should only be one ingredient on the label. The other day William picked up a tin of tomatoes and read the ingredients, expecting there to be at least 90% tomatoes. He was surprised to read that only 60% of the tins content were actual tomatoes and that the remainder, were all chemicals. This is what you are putting into your body every day.

FOODS TO AVOID

All Processed foods. They have chemicals and they contain artificial sweeteners, artificial coloring, and preservatives to add to their shelf life.

Meats	Sugars
Bacon	Anything with syrup
Burgers	Bottle/Canned Orange Juice
Chicken Wings	Cakes
Corn Beef	Candy
Liver (bad for your cholesterol)	Chocolate
Mincemeat	Cookies
Pork	Corn
Roast Duck	Desserts
Spare Ribs	Doughnuts
	Fruit Juice
	Gum
	Ice Cream
	Jams
	Jelly
	Mints
	Peanut Butter
	Sodas
	Sugar
	Pickles in Syrup

Dairy

Cheeses
Mayonnaise
Milk

Other

Canola Oil
Salad Dressing
Tin Beans
Tin Peas
Vegetable Oil

Breads, Pasta, Carbs

Bagels
Beer
Bread
Chips
French Fries
Granola
Hash Browns
Muffins
Pasta & Spaghetti
Pizza
Potatoes
Rice
Tortillas
Waffles
Wheat Based Foods
Whole Grains

Deep fried food such as those found in fast-food establishments (*you know who they are*) battered foods, breaded foods, crisps, chips, cereals, packed or tinned soups. Avoid all of these. When in a restaurant, ask them to grill your meat not fry it.

We can be fooled with sodas that say they contain minerals; we may think they are healthy when they are actually worse than beer.

If you have to drink alcohol, drink some red wine or light beer. However if you are serious about getting rid of that gut and you must have a drink, some pinot noir is okay. One to two glasses max.

SHORT TERM STRESS BUSTERS

What we are about to share will help you to cope when you feel that life is becoming too much and you begin to feel stress. You know when this happens as it is hard to sleep and difficult to relax your mind.

You will be so surprised how these little tricks can release stress and mind chatter. We only recommend what we know for certain works.

When under stress you may find it harder to eat healthy foods. In times of particularly high stress, you may eat in an attempt to fulfill emotional needs — sometimes called stress eating or emotional eating. Moreover, you may be more likely to eat processed foods even when you are not hungry.

(1) Run as fast as you can for as long as you can. You can also do this with cycling, skipping, or swimming; just give it everything you have got for a short time. Lift some weights and really do your best. Sweat it out. You will feel the change right away. Your sub-conscious will go into action to bring all systems back to a normal pace and will stop you focusing on the stress in your system.

(2) Laugh out loud while watching a very funny movie. Put a clown's nose on and look in the mirror and even walk outdoors with the clown's nose on and say hi to people. You will be uplifting other people at the same time.

(3) Listen to some great music perhaps some old disco and shake...shake...shake...that booty. Move your body in all directions. When Matthew McConaughey had to release a LOT of weight to star in Dallas Buyers Club he said he just danced all day to great music and built up a sweat to wonderful uplifting fun music. He ate smaller portions of grilled salmon or small steaks with steamed vegetables. He would still have a glass of red wine at night. He wanted to make sure he was still healthy when he lost that weight as

many actors have become quite ill after starving themselves for a movie role. He was able to gain weight after the filming and remained healthy.

(4) Stand in front of a mirror and rave about everything that you do have or the good things in your life. Do it enthusiastically and aloud. I AM so very happy and grateful for my life. My life ROCKS etc.

(5) Practice Meditation. Take three deep breaths, in through your nose and out through your mouth. Sit with your back straight for about fifteen minutes. Find some soft music with no words, (*Mozart, Beethoven etc.*) sit with your eyes closed, focus on your heart and feel the beat. If for some reason, you cannot sit just lie down on your back without a pillow and breathe.

(6) Walk on grass in your bare feet. If the grass is wet, it is even better. You can walk on sand, earth or even hug a tree. By doing this, you are grounding your body. We walk on rubber, leather as well as plastic, which can build up static in our body and when we walk barefoot, we release the electric charge. Some studies have found that grounding appears to provide some general health benefits, such as better sleep, less pain, reduced stress and better immune function.

(7) Go for a swim in the sea or a swimming pool. If that is not a possibility then have a bath or a cold shower. This is another form of grounding.

FOODS THAT HELP CALM THE MIND

Here are some great foods that can help calm your mind and let go of that stress that has been building up inside of you.

Many Yoga teachers apply these foods to their practice, to get into the flow.

Fruits & Nuts	Vegetables
Almonds	Asparagus
Avocados	Bean sprouts
Cashew nuts	Beets
Chestnuts	Broccoli
Pecans	Brussels sprouts
Sunflower seeds	Cabbage
Walnuts	Carrots
Apples	Cauliflower
Apricots	Celery
Blackberries	Cucumber
Cherries	Endive
Cranberries	Escarole
Dates	Green Beans
Figs	Jerusalem artichokes
Fresh Oranges	Kale
Grapefruit	Lentils
Grapes	Lettuce
Honeydew Melon	Parsnips
Mangoes	Quinoa
Peaches	Sweet Potatoes
Pineapple	Turnips
Plums	Watercress
Prunes	Yams
Raisins	Zucchini
Raspberries	
Tangerines (sweet)	
Watermelon	

GETTING A GOOD NIGHT'S SLEEP

Getting a good night's sleep is very important in removing and keeping the fat at bay, and due to stress and other issues going on in your life, perhaps sleep may have become a challenge.

William used to have this problem. When he was going on buying trips, he would be concerned about who will look after his business. In addition, when the containers were arriving, where to find the work force and where to store the entire product that was arriving.

He would lay awake all night with his mind racing thinking about how he was going to get through it all. When he did get to sleep, he would be dreaming about work and if he had a delivery the next day, he would be delivering the furniture in his sleep, and there were always problems in his dreams.

Even when William worked in the aviation industry, he would run a shift of about thirty plus people. He was also involved in quality control, research & development, run a JIT program, and he was responsible for the targets that had to be met each month. He was also the only one on his shift that had the certification to do X-ray, so he had to drive to a different building to do this. There was an awful amount of pressure in this job as so many were depending on him. When William left for work, he would already be tired and when he returned home, he was just plain exhausted. This was because William could not get a good night's sleep, as his mind was still at work.

Here are some suggestions that William found helped to release the stress from his work.

- Removed the TV from bedroom.

- Have a cold shower before bed.

- Tense muscles all over the body one at a time. Start with the feet and then tense for ten seconds and then relax.

- Breathing techniques, take eight deep breaths, breathe slowly in through your nose and slowly out through your mouth. So approximately, ten-seconds in, ten-second hold, ten-seconds out, ten-second hold etc.

- Remove your pillow and lie on your back. We were never meant to lie with our heads raised. This feels better for our backs.

- Avoid eating a large meal close to bedtime.

- Reduce stimulants, sugar, caffeine and alcohol.

- Use aromatherapy

- Exercise before you go to bed.

- Make your bed each morning, as a neat bed is always more appealing and helps the mind feel great and ordered when you are ready to sleep

- Make your bedroom for sleeping only, not for working on your computer.

SOME SIMPLE AND EASY WAYS TO REDUCE YOUR FAT

When you put food in your mouth, chew it 20 to 40 times.

Your stomach does not have teeth and if you do not chew your food enough, your digestive system will not be able to break it down to use it. Therefore, it will either store it as fat or just dump it.

If you do not break it down enough in your mouth, into small pieces, then your digestive system will not be able to take all the valuable contents of the food and use it to supply your body with all the important carbohydrates, proteins, fats, and nutrients that you need. If you do not do this, you will reduce the amount of nutrients you need to maintain your energy levels.

Fifty percent of your food is broken down in your mouth and not in your stomach, so keep chewing it until it is only liquid in your mouth. If you do not do this, your body will only get half of the nutrition from the food and will store a lot more fat. Plain and simple, remember that you have no teeth in your stomach. Chew your food and savor every bite. It is not a race.

No need for diet pills, simply drink lots of water.

A girl went on a diet that a health shop had advertised. She had to take this special high priced diet supplement and to stop eating six hours before she went to bed. She was told to drink lots of water during those six hours before sleep. When William met her one evening, he complemented her on how good she looked in her clothes and how great her skin looked. She then told William about her new diet and how it was worth the high price for the diet supplements.

William shared with her that he did exactly the same thing when he was training for a boxing championship, only he did NOT take diet pills and supplements he just did not eat six hours before sleep and that he drank lots of water. She was not amused, however after William explained that she could do the same thing without the high priced diet supplements and to simply experiment and see what happens. She agreed to do it because the diet supplement was very expensive.

To her great surprise, she was getting the same results without the high priced diet supplement. William saw her many times after that, she looked great and was in good shape. Too many diet gimmicks are out there and lie to you.

You may not want to do this all the time, but it is a great start and it works. Try not to eat anything for four hours before bedtime, better still if you do not eat six hours before you go to sleep. We have seen many people do this and the results are amazing. Their body size quickly becomes smaller. Of course be sensible and do not starve yourself; eat a good meal during the day. If you feel hungry, eat some of the foods we have laid out in this book to curb your appetite.

Never go hungry, ever. Keep healthy snacks like raw almonds with you at all times, when you start.

Have A Small Meal Before You Go Food Shopping.

Have a meal before you go shopping for food. If you eat before you go into the supermarket, you will not have that craving and then it is much easier to buy the food you need and not the food you crave from the senses. When you are hungry in a supermarket, your eyes and taste buds will draw you to the foods that are fatty and that contain artificial sweeteners.

They never put artificial sweeteners in good food. So eat or drink water, before you go food shopping.

Planning To Eat Out, Drink Some Water

If you are planning to eat out, drink some water and eat something light before you go to the restaurant.

Raw is best, like celery, raw almonds or cashew nuts. You will find a list of foods in this book that will take the edge off your craving. Remember the old saying; your eyes are bigger than your stomach and everything looks good on the menu when you are hungry. Most restaurants are serving foods full of artificial sweeteners and additives that are addictive. This is what makes you crave processed food even though you know that it is not good for you. It is an addiction just like a drug. Your cravings are the withdrawal symptoms of the drugs that you are putting into your body.

Even the restaurants that claim to serve healthy homemade food are generally not that healthy.

Real Lemon Juice Is Magical.

Lemon Juice/ Real Lemon is magical. When Michele would be singing at a concert for over six hours a night she would drink real lemon juice with warm water before and during breaks.

During Williams boxing days, he used to drink a glass of water with some lemon juice every hour, two weeks prior to a weigh-in.

It has to be real lemon juice and not bottled, and organic if possible. We can also do this before going to bed at night and before each meal.

It works as a detox and cleans out many of the toxins in our bodies. Lemon juice helps break down food in our stomachs for better digestion. The more efficiently our stomach breaks down food, the less work our liver has to do.

You can prepare this in the morning. Chop and squeeze a whole lemon into a liter of hot water. Then pour the contents into a glass bottle. Every hour take a drink from your bottle.

Lemons have so many benefits. It actually alkalizes your body. Lemons help break down the acidic toxins.

Here are some tips to assist in detoxing and alkalizing your organs.

- Buy a Juice Machine.
- Use fruit and vegetables. It is like a liquid diet.
- Baking Soda and Apple Cider Vinegar in water.
- Introduce one of these oils into your daily Intake. Take a tablespoon of extra virgin Olive oil every morning and night.
- Organic Udo oil, extra virgin Olive oil, Flaxseed oil, or coconut oil.
- Two tablespoons a day of these suggested oils. One tablespoon in the AM, one tablespoon in the PM.
- Drink Green tea or Oolong tea.

INGREDIENTS THAT WHEN COMBINED BURN FAT

ONLY use one of these methods DO NOT CONSUME both. In one day have one or the other. Experiment to see which one works best for your body.

Fat burning drink

Ingredients

4.6 oz of raw organic *horseradish (can be in a bottle as long as the only ingredient is horseradish)*

3 organic lemons

3 Tbl honey

2 tsp cinnamon

1 inch of raw organic ginger

Preparation

Blend 125g of horseradish and 1 piece of ginger (approx. 2cm). Take unpeeled lemons, cut them into chunks, and take out the seeds. Blend the lemon pieces together with the horseradish.

Add 3 tablespoons of honey and 2 tsp of cinnamon and stir well. Put the fat burning drink in a jar and keep it in the fridge. Take a teaspoon twice a day, along with your meals. In a matter of weeks, your waist size will reduce significantly.

Fat Burning Paste

This paste assists in Burning Fat and reduces appetite naturally.

These natural ingredients will help your body to stop storing that extra fat, and will release the fat instead.

Ingredients

Chia seeds. One and a half tablespoons

Organic Coconut oil. One tablespoon

Turmeric. One level teaspoon

Ground Cinnamon One level teaspoon

Preparation

Use a small glass or bowl. Put in your chia seeds first, then add your cinnamon, turmeric, and last add your coconut oil.

Pour enough water that is close to boiling temperature, over your ingredients. Mix until the coconut oil has turned into liquid, and has mixed thoroughly in with the rest. When cool enough eat. The coconut oil, the turmeric, and the cinnamon all are very hard to swallow, and this is why people give up on these products. When mixed with chia seeds, and the other ingredients, they lose the strength of their taste. Coconut oil is also good on its own.

Take first thing in the morning, and if you want, take it before your last meal in the evening, or as your evening meal.

BELLY FAT AND LOWER BACK PAIN

Did you know that so many people today suffer from lower back pain because of that extra bit of fat that they are carrying around on their bellies?

They spend a lot of money on painkillers, doctors, chiropractors and physiotherapists. Of course, we respect the medical profession; however, the larger percentage of people with bad backs would be just fine, if only they could release that belly fat.

Worst of all they suffer with walking, sitting, lifting, standing and sleeping. This type of pain takes control of their lives and may cause depression. People can become so focused on their pain, that it drains away all of their happiness and goodness that life can offer.

Another big surprise is that many of these people do not know the cause. They do not realize that belly fat can cause back pain, back damage and even nerve damage.

Let's look at this from a different angle. When an architect designs a two-story house, he would normally use four walls from the ground up, to support the upper part of the building. When he uses the four walls, he is distributing the weight of the upper part of the building to these four structures, and not just one.

This is the same as four people carrying a coffin. They carry it with no real problems. Now try to imagine one person trying to carry that same coffin. It would be very difficult, if not impossible.

When a tree grows, the main support is in the center, which is called the trunk of the tree. The branches grow throughout all sides of the tree, not just one side. The trunk has no real strain, as it is standing in the center and the branches balance it out.

Most people have seen forklift trucks lifting heavy loads. The person buying the forklift truck has to know the weight it will have to carry and will choose it on that basis. When the forklift truck is lifting the load in the front, the back of the truck, where the main weight is needed must be heavier. If not the truck would not be able to lift the load because the back of the truck would lift like a seesaw. Now picture your body, and see how it works.

Your spine is *not* in the center, and it is *not* on all sides. Your spine is at the back of your body, and being at the back of your body makes it a very weak structure when it comes to having to support or balance the weight of your upper body.

If you put on belly fat, that fat will pull your body forward. This puts a lot of strain on your spine. The spine has to bend forward out of its main alignment. This is where the main problem begins. Upper body fat can also cause lower back pain, as you have to carry your upper body from your lower back. So all the pressure will be on your lower back.

Another problem belly fat causes is the pulling of muscles. This can damage muscles in your lower back area, and that is very painful.

If you look at pictures of the makeup of your muscles in your body, you will see the lower back does not have many muscles in that area, and most people do not know how to work or train those muscles in this area, which are vital in supporting the upper body.

Even when you lift something with your hands, especially when your hands are out in front of your body, you are putting a lot of strain on your lower back muscles and your spine.

You can do two things to stop this type of lower back pain.

(1) Slim down and release that belly fat.

(2) Tone your stomach muscles to support your lower back.

Your stomach muscles are the main support of your upper body, for they help you lift, move or twist your upper body, and that is not all they do. Even when you lift your legs, your stomach muscles are activated. When you are climbing a ladder or climbing the stairs.

That is a great exercise for your body, running up stairs.

Have you ever seen pictures of San Francisco's Golden Gate Bridge? In photographs of this magnificent structure, you will notice how long it is, and because of the length, the bridge needs other supports to help it remain stable from its enormous weight and the San Francisco winds.

The builders of this bridge knew that this bridge could not hold its own weight. *Just like your spine trying to support your upper body.* Therefore, they built very large pillars of steel, and ran numerous steel cables from one steel pillar to the other, across the entire Bay. These steel cables had other lighter steel cables hanging down from them, and they then attach these lighter cables to the steel works on the bridge. Next, they are tightened to support the bridge.

This is the same as your spine and your lower back. You are like the steel bridge that needs that extra support. With the bridge, they used steel cables, for you a toning and strength/core building. Yes, you need to tone your stomach muscles, and then your toned stomach muscles will act like the steel cables supporting the bridge.

You muscles will support your upper body, and take the pressure off your spine and lower back. Your spine and lower back need so much extra help to support your movements of the upper body for everyday things, and especially if you need to lift anything heavy.

'12 MINUTE ABS' COOL WORKOUT

There are numerous benefits for having toned abdominal muscles and a flat belly.

The abdominal muscles, that most people call the abs, are a group of six muscles that extend from various parts of the rib area to various parts of the pelvis area. Have you heard of a great six pac? Well, you can have a great six pac!

The abdominal muscle group is a very special muscle group, because they provide postural support and movement for your upper body. Your abdominal muscles are located in your body *opposite* your lower back. This may give you incentive to release that belly fat because improving your abdominal muscles will help support your lower back and keep your body in correct alignment.

Here are just some of the benefits from toned abdominal muscles.

- Improves your back strength.
- Acts as excellent back support and improves posture.
- Can increase the efficiency of your upper body movement.
- Decreases possible back injury. Strong abdominal muscles help absorb shock during jumping, falls, running and prevents jarring motions from traveling up your body.
- Will improve your confidence, as they will make you more aware of your fitness and your body.

Most people find it almost impossible to tone up their stomach region; others simply find the exercises not very appealing. Some say that they feel the strain on other parts of their body such as their neck and back. Most of these problems occur because people think that their body is not strong or fit enough to exercise their abs, so their challenge is simply, lack of knowledge.

Michele had some issues with lower back pain from a very bad car accident she had in 1989 and was very wary of ab workouts because her body has many steel plates in her pelvis etc. Michele found Pilate's classes were safe and helped not only release all of her back pain, but also helped her have a strong core/abs. Of course, not everyone can go to Pilates so here we are going to speak about some of the easier exercises that can be done at home in front of a mirror without putting any strain on your lower back or neck.

We would have loved to have some sketches to show you however, William felt that a video would be so much better.

William decided to go to YouTube to see if there were any videos that we could recommend.

He found that so many people on YouTube were giving incorrect advice on this subject. Some were simply uploading their ego onto YouTube. They had no knowledge at all to offer, just their ego. No wonder so many people are confused about this subject, as there are so many people uploading videos with useless rubbish and speaking as if they are experts.

William finally came across an amazing person, Laura London. This woman not only knows what she is talking about, but she is living proof that it works. Laura is dedicated to helping people and the way she explains it, makes it so easy to understand.

Laura has very kindly given permission, to direct you to her YouTube video showing how to train your abs in twelve minutes standing up. This is for women and men. She shows you, and so gracefully, how to do the exercises correctly and you can work along with her.

Laura is the mother of three children and she is the real deal.

Remember your abs will not show unless you release the fat around them. You do have abs, yes you do. There is a gorgeous strong six-pac hiding under that pillow of fat. ☺

Please do not go surfing other peoples videos, stay focused on Laura's video. That is, if you want toned abs.

This is the link:

http://youtu.be/HK6mKUEY09o

AFFIRMATIONS

An affirmation is, an affirmation is, an affirmation is, yes, it is something you repeat over and over again. It is a statement of word, thought, feeling or action, which confirms a belief system or patterning that we hold in our sub-conscious mind.

Now, these can be negative or positive. It is your decision to choose negative or positive thoughts. For example, *"I am getting way too fat and I am miserable."* or, *"I am now so happy because I have started a brand new healthy life. I love to exercise my wonderful body."* Your sub-conscious mind believes everything you tell it. The sub-conscious mind is subjective. If you tell it enough, it believes and manifests that thought into your reality. Before you know it, you will be drinking lots of water and loving your healthy food choices.

GET SET now to choose only positive statements. Repeat them over and over again. Your affirmations must always be stated in the now, for the sub-conscious only knows now, and they must be personalized. If you say, *"I want to be slim, toned and healthy one day"*, your sub-conscious will NEVER know when that is going to happen. Instead say, *"I AM now at my perfect weight and I AM healthy and happy."* You see, as far as your sub-conscious is concerned, everything is NOW. So saying you want to be or you are going to be is not NOW. You must always state it in the NOW, then set your goals and be specific. Say right NOW...

I AM STRONG AND I AM HEALTHY

I LOVE TO EAT FOODS THAT ARE GOOD FOR ME

I ONLY ATTRACT GOOD IN MY LIFE

You become a magnet to what you are affirming. You become what you think about all day long. Thoughts are things. (*As you are reading this, if anything really stands out, underline it immediately. The more you understand, the more magnetic you become as your consciousness rises.*)

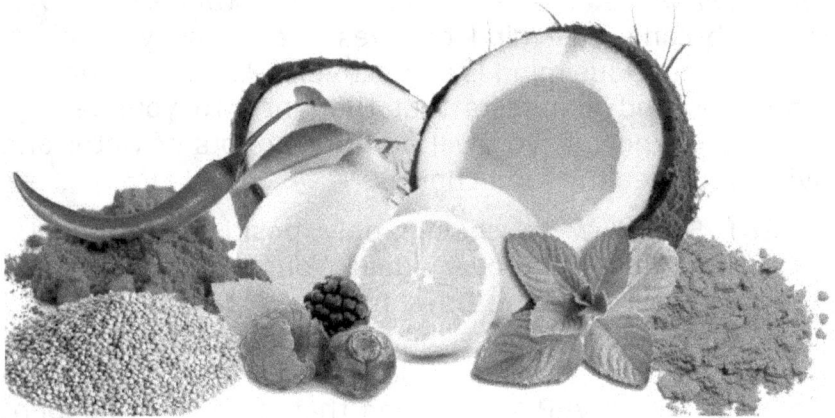

When you use positive affirmations, you are feeding your sub-conscious with positive programming or conditioning. It is simply planting good seeds of thought instead of bad. If you plant a strawberry seed, strawberries will grow. Therefore, if you plant negative thoughts, only negative conditions will grow in your experience.

Remember the sub-conscious only knows NOW. Affirmations, as with your goals, must be emotionalized, felt and believed. Become magnetic with positive thoughts. Manifest your good NOW.

Singing along to positive music is also very powerful, as you emotionalize every word through the music. Even if you are simply listening to the music, allow it to go around and around in your mind. It is similar, for example, to a cat food jingle. Instead of hearing, "I love my cat-food" (*when you may not even own a cat*), start singing to yourself:

I AM NOW AT MY PERFECT WEIGHT
LOOKING GOOD AND FEELING GREAT!

Writing down your affirmations is also very powerful, as this way you are using most of your senses. If you want, fast results write these down a minimum of fifteen times every day.

WHAT DO YOU WANT

When you begin writing, listening to and singing your affirmations, make sure you are affirming what you want and not what you DO NOT want.

Here is an example, instead of saying *"I don't want to be fat anymore"* say instead, *"I am now at my perfect weight, looking good and feeling great!"* YES, we are often repeating the same lessons, as repetition is the first law of learning and we truly wish for you to be happy, healthy and your ideal weight. We also want you to have more fun in your life. Life was not meant to be serious. Life is here to enjoy in every single magical moment. Your sub-conscious mind can be a very obedient servant when you learn how to use it for your goals and positive intentions. Be clear that what you ask for is what you truly desire. Otherwise, edit it from your mind. Next!

Next, affirmations are the foundation of your building. Think of it that way. The building is your goal. The affirmations support the building so that you can and will achieve all of your true goals. Continually feed yourself thoughts of good, build up that foundation. You deserve the best!

Say right now, *"I Will Persist Until I Succeed!"*

Be careful about what you read. Do not allow other people to do the thinking for you, for what you generally read and hear in the news is unhealthy consumption. In addition, the truth is, there is far more good than bad. If you were to interview people in the roughest and poorest neighborhood this very day, you would probably find that they had a safe and relatively trouble-free day. Most of what you read and hear in the news is magnified to sell. What do *"they"* say? Bad news sells. Good news sells, and will sell you to have a wonderful and exciting lifestyle. Only allow yourself to hear good news, read positive books, and listen to positive people and positive music.

You will find as your consciousness rises through positive thinking you will attract (*just like a magnet*) other positive people. In fact, negative people will feel uncomfortable around you. You will begin to resonate with higher vibe people.

You are a part of a universe that is abundantly unlimited. Therefore, being part of this universe, you, are abundantly unlimited. Take a look at all the stars in the sky, the leaves on the trees, and the grains of sand on the beach, plants and animal life. We are living in absolute abundance.

Look at all that nature has to offer, God does not skimp! You are surrounded in beauty and abundance. Concentrate on the beauty. When you start feeding your mind positive thoughts, you will attract creative ideas, and wonderful like-minded people. Then, the secret is to take ACTION.

LOOK AT YOUR THOUGHTS

NEVER EVER, underestimate the power of the spoken word. This may sound familiar to you. *"In the beginning was the WORD and the WORD was with God. The WORD was God. And the WORD made all things. Without the WORD was not anything made that was made."* Here the good book clearly teaches us that the physical universe is simply WORD in form. Jesus the Christ, Buddha, Paramahansa Yogananda and many other great ones said exactly the same thing, just in different ways. *"Do not judge, lest you be judged." "Love your neighbor as yourself.*

Before you can change the world, you have to change yourself. Change your thinking. We are whatever we think about all day. It is our faith that heals us. It is what we believe. *"What the mind of man can conceive and believe, he will achieve."* Napoleon Hill stated that quite clearly.

What have you been creating in your life, with your spoken word? You are the creator of all. This news is exciting! You can NOW create all good in your life. Forget about luck. You create your own so-called luck. Trust and KNOW that the universal mind, God, Christ, Buddha, or whatever you choose to call your higher power is the source of all your good. NOW let go and let God do the rest. And remember, don't take life so seriously. SMILE!

You must know at once without any doubt, that you are the one who is choosing to fear your own body and that health, fitness and happiness can be yours. It is a choice. What will you choose? Everything you created is through your previous thinking. If you want to know what thoughts, you were having yesterday, look at your life today, your body shape, your relationships, your financial situation. What will your tomorrows look like? Your body? Your relationships? Your finances? How will your life look tomorrow? It is really quite simple! You know the secret now! LOOK AT YOUR THOUGHTS TODAY. Emotions show

up in the body as physical manifestations of your thoughts.
YOU MUST CHANGE YOUR THOUGHTS.

YOU MUST BEGIN IMMEDIATELY, RIGHT NOW!

You and you alone must continually feed yourself positive thoughts. Condition yourself to a higher level of excellence every day in your life. It is like your body. You cannot begin the Ten UP System™ and in just one day expect to have a perfect body. You have to be consistent. Society may predict but only *you* can determine your own destiny. Make your own conscious decisions.

Positive changes *can* be created in mere moments. The level and emotions you feel can speed up your changes. That is why affirmations to music are so powerful. It helps to speed up the level of emotions. Will power by itself is not enough. Not if you want to achieve lasting FUN-tastic changes. Be the role model for your family and friends and everyone will want to learn your secret. You can tell them - it all started with a thought.

Every morning, as soon as you wake up, get out of bed, stretch your body and take twenty nice DEEP breaths, and then drink your water. This will help you clear your mind and body to be ready for a bright new day. Make a commitment NOW, to constantly improve yourself.

Be persistent! The magnificent spirit that you are will do anything for you however; YOU must take the first step. We are all from one Divine Mind. We are individualized creations of God. NOTHING IS IMPOSSIBLE. If one person can release weight, then so can you.

You have a lot of new programming/conditioning to feed your mind. Know, really know, that from today onwards, your life is going to improve in every area. IT IS! Speak your affirmations onto your own tape. Listen back when driving walking etc. and please, really, really feel it. Be consistent; write down your affirmations and goals. GO FOR IT!

GOAL SETTING and TAKING ACTION

First, WHAT DO YOU WANT? You cannot set your goals unless you have a clear picture of what it is that you want to achieve. This book is about releasing your body fat and/or maintaining your ideal weight, so at least you are clear on that goal. However, you can use these ideas to attract any goal you want. When you set goals, you must take action so the next section will be about how to set up blocks of time for your Daily Action List.

After you are clear about what your goals are, you must make a firm DECISION that nothing and no one is going to stop you from achieving your dreams. Not even your good self. We all have to make a Committed DECISION to have what we want!

Once a decision has been made all good will come to our aid to fulfill our goals and worthy ideals. We will be self-propelled and will find we are taking action every day to become our perfect weight looking good and feeling great. Making a decision is a real commitment and Spirit, that is us, KNOWS when we have made a real committed **YES,** to what we want.

Making a decision must never be based on *I will TRY that, but only if this happens first* etc. There are no tries, ifs or buts on the road to success and certainly not in real decision-making. If it scares us, well then we do it scared and if something does not scare and excite us at the same time then it is not a big enough dream. The things that shift our consciousness are always a little scary. This is a GOOD thing for we are growing and working outside of our old programing.

Things that before looked impossible do become possible. Do not ask how this works, MOVE and take action. Have faith in yourself and make a decision. Making a real decision will solve enormous challenges for you. Making a decision has the potential to improve almost any personal or business situation you will ever encounter and it can literally propel you down the path to incredible success.

The world's most successful people share a common quality. They make decisions and rarely if ever change their minds. Yes, decision makers go to the top and those who do not make decisions seem to go nowhere. Think about it...

The health of your mind and body, the well-being of your family, your social life, the type of relationships you develop, are all-dependent upon your ability to make sound decisions. Most of us will not often make decisions on our own, many individuals look first to see what others will think of their choices. This is not freedom. ONLY YOU know what you want so only YOU can be the one making decisions about your own life. As long as what you decide is not harming yourself or others GO FOR IT. Especially if what you want is helping you become healthier and is educating your mind and spirit then say YES to what you want to achieve.

No one but YOU knows what is best for you.

Do not make your decisions and then worry about whether you are doing the right thing. Especially when it comes to your health and fitness, it is important to understand that it is not difficult to learn. With the proper information and by subjecting yourself to certain disciplines we are sharing in this book, you can become a very proficient and effective decision maker.

You can virtually eliminate conflict and confusion in your life by becoming proficient in making decisions. Decision-making brings order to your mind. Moreover, of course, this order is reflected in your objective world, your results.

No one can see you making decisions, but they can always see the *results* of your decisions. When after one or two months of working with the TEN UP SYSTEM™ and you see old friends, do not be surprised if they do not recognize you. For you will have not only changed on the outside also your inner vibration and confidence will be obvious.

Therefore, make decisions based on what YOU WANT and then do not change your mind and do not let outside appearances or other people influence you.

REMEMBER YOUR THOUGHTS ARE POWERFUL

Make a Decision and go for it...

You also have to be consistent in your workouts and persistent. **Whatever you can conceive and believe, through persistence, you must achieve.**

Make persistence your most well developed mental muscle. Persistence cannot be replaced by any other quality. Superior skills will not make up for it. A well-rounded, formal education cannot make up to replace it. Nor will calculated plans nor a magnetic personality. When you are persistent, you will become your perfect weight looking good and feeling great.

The most powerful speech ever given was by the world-renowned orator Sir Winston Churchill and the whole speech consisted of only three words.

Never Give Up! Never Give Up! Never Give Up!

Churchill knew what that really meant. He had a whole nation relying on him during the Second World War.

How do you become persistent?

You are not born with it and you cannot inherit it. There is no one in the entire world that can develop persistence for you. Ultimately, persistence becomes a way of life, but that is not where it begins. To develop the mental strength, *persistence*, you must first really want something. You have to want something so much that it becomes a heated desire, a passion.

You must fall in love with the idea of being fit, healthy and having longevity. You must fall in love with the idea. You have to magnetize yourself to every part of the idea. Then persistence will be automatic. The very idea of not persisting will become hateful and anyone who even attempted to take your dream away from you, stop you, or slow you down would be in serious trouble. Difficulties, obstacles, and mountains will appear in one form or another and sometimes our own minds will make molehills into mountains but because of persistence, they will be defeated every time. Make a statement to the treasury of your sub-conscious mind, as if what you really want has already happened. You write out, what you want to happen in your life the night before, but you write it in a way, as to state that this event has happened and you are now saying thank you for it happening, and you are living it right now in your life.

You can do it in the morning, at night, and repeat the statement in your head during the day with feeling.

The statement should go like this.

EXAMPLE

I GIVE THANKS THAT I AM NOW in the best shape of my life, and I have so much energy and yet I feel peaceful and calm. I am wearing the size clothes that I always wanted to wear, and I am wearing the body I always wanted to experience. I FEEL GREAT!

Every morning you write down your goals and remember to feel gratitude.

CREATING A MAGNETIC FUTURE SELF BOARD

Vision boards have been used in the personal development area for many years now. Vision boards have even been featured on Oprah and Ellen, and you probably have heard of vision boards as a great way to graphically illustrate your hopes and dreams, as well as increase the likelihood that you will get what you want.

A vision board has images stuck on to a board that are a visual representation of things that you want in your life, things that you believe will make you happier. It consists of a board, which can be made from various materials like cardboard with cut out pictures that would be selected by you.

The purpose of this is for you to convince your sub-conscious mind, that your reality is what is on the board in these pictures.

The mechanics of creating a vision board is quite simple and easy. You get a piece of poster board or some cardboard, scissors, some glue or pins, and some magazines. You can be as creative as you like, as this is for you and only you. Make sure that each picture on your vision board evokes a positive emotional response from you. Just looking at your vision board will make you feel good and more positive.

Place you vision board in a place where you are getting maximum exposure to it. Constantly bathe your sub-conscious mind with the images and statements on this board. Place the vision board in a place where it is private for you.

Get some magazines, like fashion or holiday magazines, and cut out the pictures you like. Pictures of places you would like to visit, and if you see someone that is the perfect size and weight, that you would like to be, cut out that picture and then cut out from one of your photographs your own smiling face on that body. Put as many pictures as you like up on your vision board.

Next, write statements in the NOW just the way you did with your affirmations. Statements like, I AM so happy and I AM so grateful now that I AM at my perfect weight looking good and feeling great! Read these statements and at the same time gaze at your vision board. Take it all in and feel the happy emotions that you would have when you are, that perfect body size. This is very important. Do this as many times a day as possible. The most powerful time to do this is just before you go to bed at night and when you first wake up in the morning.

Your sub-conscious mind works in images and patterning. When you are looking at these pictures and reading the statements regularly, your sub-conscious mind will start to believe that this is your reality right now. This will attract the right people and circumstances into your life to create this new reality. You can use this in many areas of your life.

Do not get frustrated that you do not have what you want right this moment. Never give up and always feel gratitude. Gratitude is a very vital part of creating your new life. Do your best to detach yourself from the outcome. Just enjoy the feelings you are experiencing when you are looking at your vision board. At first, you may have some difficulty visualizing, that is okay. A great tool that will really help you is something Michele created back in 1993 and has named **The Magnetic Future Self Board.**

Go ahead and make the DECISION to have what you desire. No matter what your present circumstances, your good WILL appear. In fact, what you desire also desires you. At the right place and the right time, you will find each other. Whatever your good is this is your time to DREAM BIG DREAMS!

NOW MOVE! DO IT! Make it colorful and have fun.

This picture is an example of a
vision board Michele created.
Inside of the magnet you tape your pictures.

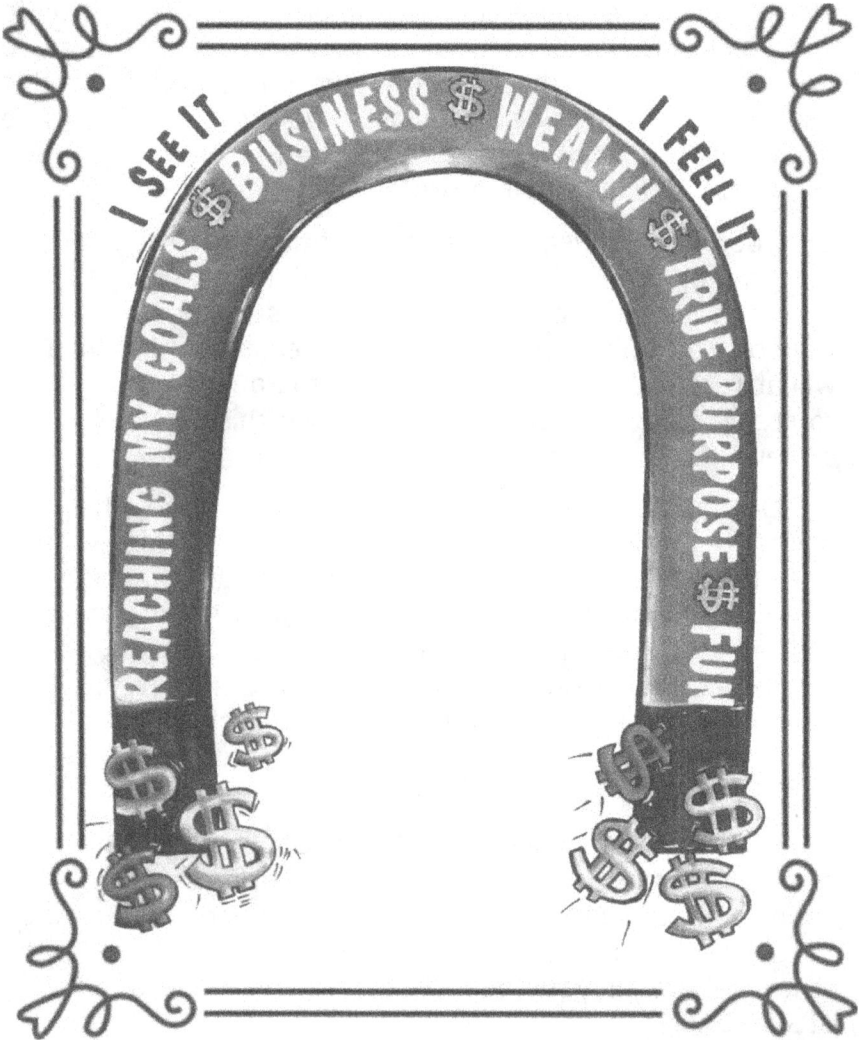

YOUR DAILY ACTION LIST!

It has been proven in many research studies that people who write down their goals DO achieve them and when we add the power of the mind, decision and persistence with a planned daily action list, well then, you will become a legend in your own life. It seems so simple, however not many people will stick to a plan or even write down any goals. Create a BIG GOAL and every day you work, follow a positive action list. Be one of the 3% group who NEVER GIVES UP.

When you first begin doing a daily action list you will find that projects in the past that seemed impossible to complete will now be completed and *ahead of time.* Your life will begin to have clarity and order and your success will begin flowing. You will be able to accomplish more with less time. No more doing things just to be busy. Doing this list WILL help you in ways that will seem miraculous.

Instructions

Write down your daily action list at night. You will do your daily list every evening for thirty days. Why write your list in the evening? Because as you are sleeping your sub-conscious mind will help you attract opportunities and creative ideas, for those actions to come to fruition. It will help you be self-propelled to take positive, enthusiastic action the next day.

Tape your action list up on a wall where you work each day and highlight each action that is completed with a bright yellow highlighter after each is completed. We recommend you write down the hardest action first. You will find that making that call you have been putting off early in the morning after you have meditated and completed your workout and spiritual practices will no longer scare you. Doing the actions that you do not like or that intimidate you *first* will help you gain light and power. *You know* those things that you keep putting off.

Research has proven that doing this will accelerate your goals into action faster than you could ever imagine. You will no longer be a procrastinator; you will be a doer not a wishful thinker. Of good, will begin to appear in your life. If you have not completed the six items on your list by the end of the evening, add what was not completed to the next day's list. Do not beat yourself up too much (*maybe a little bit* ☺) if you haven't done them all. Say to yourself, *"This is so simple. It is worth it to me. I will have clarity. I will know what I've done. I will stay clear. I will be getting things done that are helping me achieve my dreams towards a slim, toned, healthy body and my success in life. I am committed to taking these positive actions on my daily action list. I know that each detail is just as important as any other."*

You know the saying, *"God is in the details"*! Do each action with total focus and impeccability. Doing each action with love, focus and impeccability will also keep you mindful. If you find you are not doing all of the things on your DAILY LIST, perhaps you have put up one action step that is too big to be one action. **This is not goal setting; these are actions to help you complete your goals.**

You don't list a project/goal as one item on your DAILY LIST. Instead, break it down into doable action steps.

By breaking down your goals into manageable pieces, you will find that your six actions will be very easy to do. DO NOT overwhelm yourself by putting more than six items on your DAILY LIST. Just do one thing at a time.

The reason we have indicated a numbered day *(thirty in total)* for each DAILY LIST is because you will want to make sure that you do this list every single day for a full consecutive thirty days. That is right, seven days a week. This way it will become an easy thing to do and will no longer feel like a discipline. It will be just as easy as brushing your teeth and showering. It will become a new positive habit. After the initial thirty days, you can do four or five days a week if that is what you choose to do, however doing this list for the first time in a consecutive thirty days, will create an amazing NEW Habit, a new Positive Paradigm and increase your clarity and your results exponentially. You will FEEL SO GOOD about yourself *because* YOU DID IT!

If you do miss a day, you have to start over from day one. Even if it is at day twenty-five, if you miss one day, you have to begin at Day One until a full thirty days is completed. You may be up to day twenty-eight and miss it because of just feeling like you deserved a day off, however that is simply your old paradigm clicking back in again, so forgive yourself and begin again at day one. Soon this will become a new habit that you will find gives you deep satisfaction and fulfillment. Yes, you WILL see definite positive results. You will know that this initial thirty days was well worth it as you will be so ahead in the game of life that it will literally feel miraculous. You can do this. Do it for you!

Please do not cheat by making any justifications; there is no point in cheating yourself that is just silly. This is YOUR LIFE and YOU are the one who is responsible for making YOUR LIFE WORK.

You deserve this for you!

So be excited and begin DAY ONE of your daily action list. We suggest you add one more thing to your list. *Today I serve another.* This can be through a tithe, an act of kindness, a gift, a smile to a stranger etc. When you think of others, life is so much sweeter and rewarding.

The next page is a sample of a daily action list...

~ **MY DAILY LIST** ~

for:_____

I am so excited about becoming focused and doing my positive daily action list because I KNOW that taking these actions are definitely helping my dreams come true and I AM becoming my perfect weight as I exercise my body with joy and gratitude every day.

I LOVE doing these positive actions. It is easy for me to do my daily list, one positive action at a time.

Positive Action #1

Positive Action #2

Positive Action #3

Positive Action #4

Positive Action #5

Positive Action #6

The Power Of Meditation

Practicing Meditation forms a most important part of our work in becoming a healthy, disciplined calm and successful person. You will have clarity, love and peace of mind. The reason we say practicing, is because Eternity meditates us...we call it practicing meditation until we have the real experience of total oneness.

Now because the purpose of this book is to give you tools to assist you in becoming fit, toned, and happy through releasing unhealthy, unwanted fat, we are not going to go too deeply into what the Power of Meditation truly is. If you wish to know more of the mystical side, you can always visit Michele's website. www.MysticalSuccessClub.com. On her site, Michele has loads of free videos that cover many mystical topics including; How to Practice Meditation and how to discover your true-life purpose.

Why meditate? Because if we desire to truly move ahead and have health, vitality and energy we must tap into that which sustains all. If we wish to truly connect with our higher self and not get into thinking it is our own mind that is creating or attracting what we want then this chapter on meditation will assist you to look more deeply. This chapter will teach those who have never meditated before and will remind those who do practice meditation, its' awesome power. When we practice meditation, we are consciously connecting, in the silence, to our Higher Power.

Although there are many ways taught to achieve silence through meditation practice, we will share with you some ideas that will meet your needs very nicely.

Create your own space where you will meditate. Clean this area thoroughly, as this will release old lines of energies because when we meditate it is best to have clean energy. Buy a brand new mat on which to sit. Light a beautiful candle, as you can use the candle flame to focus your attention. A candle *does* bring good energy into your space as does traditional incense. A flower or some kind of lush green plant is also good. If you do not live alone, ask your roommate or partner to please respect that this is your special place. Of course, to actually sit outdoors on the earth is always wonderful but always designate a special place where you live to meditate and please meditate alone. Do not meditate in your bed as you will add too much energy to your bed and you may find it difficult to sleep because meditation gives us more energy. Meditation is not meant to make you sleepy; it is a much-focused practice. Visualization exercises are OK to do in bed as you can then flow into a positive sleep, filled with pictures of you at your perfect weight, happy and calm. You can take these beautiful images into your dream plane.

Once you have your meditation space prepared and cleaned sit down on your mat (*lotus style if you can*) sit up straight, arms out to your sides and breathe in through your nose deeply, hold it and then exhale slowly through your mouth. Keep doing this until you feel peaceful. As you are now sitting quietly, place your attention centered somewhere between the eyes and a little above, and take some word that is powerful to you, you will know it when you try some words out. LOVE, BLISS, GOD, SPIRIT, BEAUTY and ponder the word you choose. Some lovely mantra's are, *As a wave is one with the ocean I am One with God, As a ray of light is one with the sun I am one with God, I Love God, or God's Grace is flowing through me, I am now a clear instrument for God's Grace,* or *Om Mani Padme Hum* or just the word *OM.* Use only one power word if that suits you better. You do not have to be religious to do this. This is about focus and connection and meditation practice *will* strengthen your mind. Replace the word God with Love, if this feels more comfortable.

As you are sitting and focused on your power word, Love, Heart etc. your thoughts *will* wander off, when this happens gently refocus your mind back to the same mantra or word. Feel no impatience with yourself or frustration. No matter how many times your mind wanders, bring it back to that one word.

If you do this simple method, eventually, you will find that annoying intruding thoughts will cease, and you will be able to sit quietly in a peaceful state. It may take days or it may take weeks to acquire this steadiness of mind, but it will come if you have patience and are consistent.

At first, do not attempt to remain quiet for more than five minutes or so unless you feel like it. After a couple of weeks meditate for ten minutes and so on, until you can sit comfortably for much longer periods. We are doing this to have a conscious realization of our unity with Spirit or to make contact with God. There are no bad meditations, each intention to sit and quietly connect to our Divine Source, eventually *will* awaken us from the sleep of life to our higher consciousness.

We are not attempting to see "light" or to have "experiences". If they do come just refocus the mind, as if we become too fascinated with these "experiences" we could lose sight of the original intention and make way too much of them. Keep it simply. KISS – "Keep It Simple and Spiritual", and remember to smile as we wish to bring a happy vibration to our meditation time. You can name it your *Happy Meditation*.

After we have had a few minutes of meditation and have achieved that feeling of peace, joy and unity with the Universe give thanks, get up and go about our day. It is recommended that we do this three or four times a day. First thing in the morning, at lunchtime (*noon until two pm is best*) and then at night (*best when sun is setting a powerful time to connect with God's presence*) and then at midnight or just before we are to go to bed.

When we first begin this practice, perhaps just meditate for five minutes three times a day or for some

145

perhaps just having the intention to connect with your soul for two – three minutes say four or five times a day will help. This will be a great start.

Why?

Ultimately, meditating three or four times a day even if for just a few minutes each time, will bring us to a place where we will be focused and unified with the Divine Presence all day, whether asleep or awake.

Even if you are agnostic, look at meditation as physicians do. It has been documented that people who meditate regularly have low blood pressure and generally are healthier, happier human beings. So do it, even if the word God is not your thing. Put a smile on your face as you sit down to meditate as this DOES help your mind find peace. Do whatever you can to put yourself into a happy mindset before you sit down.

As mentioned, this chapter is a simple way of learning to practice meditation. Before we truly experience real silence, we are all only practicing meditation. However, every time we do this we DO raise our consciousness, even if we do not realize it. In time, we will feel better and clearer and definitely less clogged or stressed. It is NOT to be taken in an overly serious tone, focused yes, but not so serious. Oscar Wilde said, *"Life is too serious to be taken seriously,"* so LIGHTEN UP! Focus your attention and feel happiness and gratitude. This way it is a simple and easy way to begin to practice, but do not underestimate its power. If you do not at first FEEL any connection or peace of mind that is OK. Just having the intention to consciously connect and feel the presence of God will eventually create in you, peace, joy and everything good will begin flowing your way.

WHY?

Because at least for a few minutes a day you have chosen to get out of the way and let God in. As you delve into longer meditations and find a way that suits you best, and there are many different ways to learn meditation, your life and physical well-being WILL radically change for the better. Oh yes it will.

If you are having a challenge with your meditation practice, do not give up; allow these loving and all wise words by the great soul Paramahansa Yogananda to assist you, "*Your trouble with meditation is that you don't persevere long enough to get results. That is why you never know the power of a focused mind. If you let muddy water, stand still for a long time, the mud will settle at the bottom and the water will become clear. In meditation, when the mud of your restless thoughts begins to settle, the power of God begins to reflect in the clear waters of your consciousness. You will become a smile millionaire.*"

Yes, let us all become Smile Millionaires! Always remember to smile sincerely and breathe...Life is magical, oh yes, it is!

Love And Gratitude

The power of Love and Gratitude is something that only a few people are aware of and even fewer people understand that it is the true path to happiness. There are people on the planet today that heal with love and gratitude. To be happy, you must know what happiness is and what it is not. People tend to confuse happiness with the causes of happiness. For example, you are happy when you hold a kitten or a cute puppy, when your team wins. However, these are all causes and therefore they are only temporary forms of happiness.

Happiness is a journey, not a destination. Happiness means you have an overall feeling that life is going well. Happiness does not mean you have to be an outwardly enthusiastic person, as a very happy person may be very up vibe or very quiet. Positive emotions come from gratitude. Doing what you say you are going to do and doing your actions with love.

You can increase your peace and happiness greatly by taking some time to write to other people and thank them for being in your life. (*A letter or card NOT email*) Another very powerful exercise is to write yourself a letter. Yes, write yourself a gratitude letter and then mail it to yourself. Do this regularly. You do not expect to maintain your perfect weight by just one day of exercise etc. so this too is something to maintain regularly, your gratitude.

People can change everything in their lives by applying love and gratitude.

Just listen to your heart and you will know what the truth is. All we ask from you is to keep an open mind.

Dr Masaru Emoto is a doctor of Alternative Medicine who has authored books on the effects of water when exposed to love and gratitude. He took pictures of the frozen samples. He also took pictures of samples that were not exposed to love and gratitude. As we do not have permission to duplicate his photos, we suggest you look him up or watch a short video on YouTube that shows how words and intention GREATLY affect water.

https://www.youtube.com/watch?v=iu9P167HLsw

About seventy percent of the human body is made up of water and, coincidentally, more than seventy percent of Earth is covered in water. Fatty tissue contains less water than lean tissue. Very interesting!

Obesity decreases the percentage of water in the body, sometimes to as low as forty five percent. So drink lots of water and you will have more Divine Water to bless your being.

Remember your body is made of approximately seventy percent water. Remember this and LOVE your body. Love your Life. BE GRATEFUL.

Putting It All Together

Now, that you have read our book, we would love you to continue your journey and discover the awesome power you have inside of you. If you only knew the knowledge and information and power that is inside of you, and has been waiting for this moment, for you to set it free, you would be in ecstatic gratitude.

You are like an iceberg, but all this time you have been focused on the little bit of you that is above the water surface, and unaware of the huge part that is beneath the surface. The funny thing is, that huge part is the real you.

One of the best ways to move forward from here is to train with the Ten UP System™ three times a week and on the other four days go for a walk, get on a treadmill or do some yoga or Pilates on the other days. Remember the idea here is to use the Ten UP System™ to create the body we know you have always wanted.

This is it.

1. When you awake in the morning drink two pints of water.

2. Read your list that you wrote the night before.

3. Visualization for five minutes.

4. Practice of meditation.

5. Write out your Goals.

6. Picture all that is good in your life and rave about it.

7. Practice your Affirmations.

8. Focus your thoughts on what you want in your life, not on what you do not want.

9. If you catch yourself thinking about what you don't want. Just say in your mind. NEXT. Then refocus on what you do want.

10. Watch what you talk about to others.

11. Acknowledge your mind and ask it to give you solutions to any challenge or any inquiry about your life. If you ask your mind/spirit before you go to bed, you will wake up with the answers. Your spirit is magical and loves you.

12. Stay away from the news.

13. Exercise and do some stretching.

14. Drink lots of water all day.

What others are saying about The Mystical Success Club™...

"Michele Blood is truly a special person. For over three decades, I have made serious study of the mind and how to live a full and balanced life. I have taught tens of thousands of people around the world how to properly utilize their God-given potential, and then along came Michele Blood. She had a very positive impact on my life, for which I am truly grateful! She made me aware of unique methods for realizing more power by effectively combining affirmations and music. Invest in her entire library and let this petite powerhouse show you a fast and effective way to enjoy more of life's rich rewards. I enthusiastically introduce Michele Blood and her wonderful work to every audience. Order her material today! Share Michele and MusiVation™ discovery with your world; they will thank you with sincere gratitude." **- Bob Proctor, Author of the Best Selling Book "You Were Born Rich"**

Michele belongs in every achiever's library.

- Samuel A. Cypert, Author of "Achieve & Believe"

Dearest Michele, I want to say Thank You So Much for all that you are doing for the Mystical Club Members. You have made my life alive again. Thank you, Thank you...- **Patti C**

Being introduced to Michele's Mystical Success Club my life has changed for the best. I can get the most powerful, up-lifting and energizing emotions when I participate in any of Michele's in-person or Weimar sessions. My life has been so hectic over the past few months, but I make it my priority to spend time listening and learning from Michele, because she brings my life back into absolute consciousness. I appreciate and treasure the time Michele dedicates to helping those who are searching for their higher self. I absolutely feel I achieve a higher consciousness with each and every one of Michele's sessions. Thank you, thank you, thank you.... I am gaining momentum to my higher self, to reaching my unlimited consciousness. God Bless You Michele. - **Don Runowski**

When Michele first prayed for me and gave me specific instructions to feel the stillness within I was in over $500,000 credit card debt in just 4 months I was out of debt through a totally unexpected gift. I feel free and happy and am now in a new Beautiful relationship with someone who really gets me. - **J'En El Author/speaker**

We Highly Recommended These Two Books

"The Coconut Oil Miracle" by Bruce File

"Become A Magnet To Money Through The Sea Of Unlimited Consciousness" (2 Books In One) by Bob Proctor and Michele Blood

Write Out Your Goals and Positive Intentions

Write Out Your Goals and Positive Intentions

Write Out Your Goals and Positive Intentions

Write Out Your Goals and Positive Intentions

Write Out Your Goals and Positive Intentions

www.ingramcontent.com/pod-product-compliance
Lightning Source LLC
Chambersburg PA
CBHW072011290326
41934CB00007BA/1055